THE COMPLETE GUIDE TO
YIN YOGA

The Philosophy and Practice of Yin Yoga

BERNIE CL
FOREWORD BY SARAH

WILD STRAWBERRY PRODUCTIONS
VANCOUVER, B.C. CANADA

This book was originally published by White Cloud Press.

Cover and interior design by Confluence Book Services

First edition: 2011

Printed in the Unites States

2019 2018   14 13

Library of Congress Cataloging-in-Publication Data
Clark, Bernie, 1953-
The complete guide to yin yoga : the philosophy and practice of yin yoga / by Bernie Clark.
    p. cm.
Includes bibliographical references and index.
ISBN 978-1-935952-50-3 (pbk.)
1. Yin yoga. I. Title.
 RA781.73.C53 2011
 613.7'046--dc23
                    2011028908

Credits for Art and Photography

Chapters 2, 3, & 4: Photographs of Cherise Richards, our Yin Yoga model, are by Christy Collins. Copyrighted 2011 by Bernie Clark.

Chapter 6: p. 195: "The Myofascial-Tendon Complex," reprinted, by permission, from SEER Training Modules, Structure of Skeletal Muscle. U. S. National Institutes of Health, National Cancer Institute. <http://training.seer.cancer.gov/anatomy/muscular/structure.html>; p. 196: "Collagen Fibers," reprinted, by permission, Matthew P. Dalene and the Rensselaer Plytechnic Institute; p. 201: "Connective Tissues," reprinted from *Gray's Anatomy, 38th Edition, The Anatomical Basis of Medicine and Surgery Copyright*, p. 76, by Pearson Professional Limited 1995 and with their kind permission; p. 208: "Types of Synovial Joints," reprinted, by permission, Produnis of the Wikimedia Share Commons.

Chapter 7: p. 256: "The Cell's Cytoskeleton" from *Energy Medicine–The Scientific Basis*, p. 46, copyright Elsevier Limited, 2000, reprinted, by permission, from Elsevier and James Oschman.

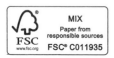

For Nathalie, who has come to share in my belief that yin is truly in!

Table of Contents

Foreword

The practice of yoga has always been evolving, but essentially yoga is the cultivation of attention. What we attend to and the attitude with which we attend greatly influence how we experience ourselves and our life. In yoga we concentrate on both form (our bodies and tissues), and formlessness (our breath, energy channels, and mind states). These interconnected aspects of reality are in constant interplay, they are the Yin and Yang of life, and, in yoga we develop and balance these polar complementarities within our body/mind experience. For most of us, beginning with that which is most tangible, the body (Yang) is a common doorway into the practice. As we become less distracted and healthier physically, most students eventually become interested in that which is more hidden. This can be called the yin aspect of reality, which relates with that which is subtle. It is only by paying attention in a relaxed and attuned way that this yin aspect of yoga is revealed.

When students first begin a yoga practice, perhaps to reduce stress or to get in shape, or maybe just to accompany a friend, they will often be guided to place the largest percentage of their attention on the shape of the poses they are trying to do. This keeps the practice safe and as we learn postural integration, our body-based experience becomes more joyous, healthy, and the postures more fun to inhabit. Eventually, with skillful guidance, sincere practitioners become interested not only in the outer forms of yoga, but in the inner revolution that yoga can offer, or, as Bernie might say, they start to go *yin-side*. It is here that the deeper aspects of yoga are revealed.

Paying attention to the fluctuations of the breath, noticing the sensations ebbing and flowing in the physical body, tracking the changing feelings in the emotional body, and recognizing the space of the mind as well as the thoughts in the mental body are all part of yoga. This yoking or joining of the body, heart, and mind provides health benefits beyond simply being more flexible or stronger. The word *health* is derived from an Old English word meaning "whole." Yoga re-establishes our natural wholeness — the balanced integrity of our yin and yang nature.

Adding a yin or quieter aspect to our yoga practice can introduce us to the possibility of physical/emotional/mental equilibrium by marrying the softer, contemplative modes of being in life to the stronger activities we are so often compelled by. This helps reduce the compulsive extremes of behavior that cause us to lose balance, lose focus, and diminish our joy of living. Yang energy is needed to bring vitality to our yin interior, but it is the gentler yin qualities within us that balance our yang intensities. If you have felt that life is too often not how you would like it to be, then learning the ancient art of deep listening, tuning in to the internal, non-conceptual, softer aspects of your yin nature may be the healing direction.

Yin Yoga, when taught skillfully, can provide this opportunity to go within and re-align our orientation. It will also affect our physical body in ways that may surprise us. It is simple, but often challenging. It will provide us with ample periods of stillness within which we can start to pay attention to what is really happening, right here, right now. It can provoke insights that may move us to make significant changes in our life or allow us to accept that what is happening right now is exactly what ought to be happening right now. We may discover ourselves opening up to and connecting with our experience as it is, rather than holding on to resistance and feelings of victimization.

For anyone seeking to learn and benefit from the practice of yoga, this book will be an invaluable guide. Bernie has been a student and friend of mine for many years. I know him to be a thoughtful and dedicated teacher who has helped many through his workshops, website, and writings. Through this book, he is sharing his own practice for all our benefits, seeking to help anyone who desires genuine health and wholeness. Within these pages, you will find explorations on the physical benefits of Yin Yoga and explanations on the ways Yin Yoga helps us energetically as well as emotionally and mentally. The practice of Yin Yoga is described in detail and the various *asanas* are reviewed in a simple way, allowing them to be fully experienced. For those interested, the evolution of yoga in general and Yin Yoga specifically is also presented.

It is with heartfelt encouragement that I invite you to experience opening within through the study and practice of Yin Yoga.

Sarah Powers
New York
September 2011

Preface

Many readers of my previous book, *YinSights: A Journey into the Philosophy & Practice of Yin Yoga*, wrote to tell me how much they enjoyed reading it and how valuable they found the practice of Yin Yoga. Along with many emails, there were also requests posted in the YinYoga.com Forum asking for even more information: how to get into the poses described in the book and how to safely come out of them, how to do Yin Yoga for the upper body, whether Yin Yoga would be helpful for unique, special situations, and lots of other questions. Many readers asked about the Daoist history that also informed and influenced the development of Yin Yoga. The demand grew for a second edition of YinSights that would cover these and other details of the practice of Yin Yoga.

Unfortunately, a technical challenge arose: adding to the information already presented in *YinSights* would make the book unwieldy. *YinSights* was already over 400 pages long and extending it to answer all the questions being raised would make the book too bulky. A second edition did not seem like a good idea. Fortunately the opportunity arose to solve this problem by creating, not a second edition of *YinSights* but a new book focused more tightly on the practice of Yin Yoga and its benefits and less on the philosophy and evolution of yoga in general. The result is what you are reading right now.

The Complete Guide to Yin Yoga borrows heavily in many places from *YinSights*, but it extends what was presented in the earlier book considerably. Yinsters familiar with *YinSights* will find a few sections repeated entirely but they will also find an expanded description of the Yin Yoga postures, more flows following broader themes, and postures designed to work the upper body. Special situations are also covered, such as how to modify your Yin Yoga practice if you are pregnant or what to do to help you become pregnant. There is a more complete examination of the effects of Yin Yoga on our fascia and also on our muscles too.

Of course the benefits of Yin Yoga go far beyond the physical, and this book will also describe the considerable mental, emotional and energetic benefits we can receive through the practice of Yin Yoga. I hope previous readers will enjoy *The Complete Guide to Yin Yoga* as much as they did *YinSights* and that new readers will be inspired to take a walk on the yin-side. After all, yin is in!

Acknowledgements

Showing the way fearlessly and compassionately,
the stream of all our Ancestral Teachers,
to whom we bow in gratitude.
From *Touching The Earth*, A *gatha* of the
monastics of Plum Village, France

Writing a book begins as a solitary endeavor, but never one that starts without encouragement. Along the way, through all the stops and starts, friends appear who give us the strength to continue. There are many people I wish to thank for helping make this guide a reality. Firstly, I would like to thank Steve Scholl and Paul Grilley for suggesting the project in the first place. Of course I would not even be in a position to write about Yin Yoga if it were not for all my teachers, to whom I bow in gratitude.

My eternal thanks to my first Yin Yoga teacher, Sarah Powers, who helped me understand how to slow down and mindfully practice yoga. *Pranams* to Paul Grilley who introduced me to so many of the concepts presented in this book; to Jim Clark, for keeping me straight on the science.

I would also like to single out the White Cloud Press team who contributed so importantly to the work: to Raina for her tireless and excellent editing, to Christy Collins for her photography, design and layout, to Cherise Richards for posing again and again, and to Stephen Sendar and Steve Scholl for their patience. I thank also Pilar Wyman for her indexing help.

Finally, my blessings and thanks to all the students who have allowed me the honor of teaching them: the best way to learn a subject is to try to teach it. Indeed, my students have been my greatest teachers.

▷▷▷**Please Note!** Before embarking on this practice, please make sure you are able to do so: check with your doctor or health care professional before starting any yoga practice. The guidance given in this book is not meant to replace medical advice and should be used only as a supplement if you are under the care of a health care professional. While care has been taken in compiling the guidance in this book, we cannot take any responsibility for any adverse effects from your practice of yoga. When you are not sure of any aspect of the practice, or feel unwell, seek medical advice. Please read the contraindications for each pose before you try the pose, so that you will know if this particular posture is a good one for you to try. Be aware of the many options available to make each pose more accessible. Practice with both intention and attention.

Introduction

Modern yoga has sprung from a figurative forest of many different styles of yoga with many varied intentions. In the earliest records of ancient India, yogis were mythical beings with powers that could transcend this physical realm. One particular tree germinating in this fertile forest about 1,000 years ago is called Hatha Yoga, which means the forceful yoga. Hatha Yoga, distinct from the other trees in the yoga forest, was primarily designed to strengthen the body and prepare it for other forms of yoga; these forms could be the meditative practices that lead to liberation and enlightenment but Hatha Yoga could also be a path towards developing darker arts and black magic. Many Hatha yogis were famed for their prowess as warriors and were hired as mercenaries.

Today, we mostly know of Hatha Yoga in the West as the practice that makes us healthier and calmer. Not too many practitioners of yoga today are aiming for spiritual awakening, although if that happens, that might be nice. The intentions for attending a yoga class today may range from seeking health to seeking companionship. The fact that you can actually take a yoga class today is very new: there were no classes in ages past—you learned by sitting at the feet of your guru. If you were lucky, he would impart to you everything he learned from his guru, but this transmission would take many long years of dedicated study and practice.

The Hatha tree sprouted many stout branches. Far more than the physical postures, or asanas, the original practice emphasized the breath and magic circles formed by the hands and body, called mudras. In the last 100 years, asanas have moved into the spotlight in the evolving Western versions of Hatha Yoga. There are dozen of branches now: some of the oldest are called Ashtanga Yoga, Iyengar Yoga, and Sivananda Yoga while some of the newest and smallest shoots have names like aqua yoga, dance yoga and wine & chocolate yoga. Most of these modern forms of Hatha Yoga emphasize health and wellness physically, mentally and emotionally.

With the modernization of Hatha Yoga, some things have been lost. The original forms of Hatha Yoga equally emphasized strong muscular activities, which can be characterized as yang practices, and the softer activities that opened our deeper tissues such as the joints, which can be characterized as the yin practices. The yin-side of yoga is found now only hidden inside a few softer styles such as restorative yoga and in the meditation practices, which very few people are drawn to. This is an unfortunate omission because it robs the student of the chance to develop enhanced health for the whole body, heart and mind.

This book is an investigation into that missing half: Yin Yoga. The investigation will take you into the philosophical underpinnings of yin versus yang and will explain the benefits of adding a yin perspective to your yoga practice. These benefits are considerable and are found in all aspects of our life: from our physical well-being to our mental and emotional well-being.

The practice of Yin Yoga is explained here in detail, but a book is never a substitute for a teacher. If you are drawn to investigate this part of the Yoga forest further, you are encouraged to seek out a Yin Yoga teacher that you can relate to. Like all yoga practice, theory alone is insufficient: you must actually do the practice. It is entertaining and educational to read about how and why you might do Yin Yoga, but the real value comes in actually getting down on the floor. So...as you begin to read this book, get off your couch, get out of your chair, place a cushion on the floor and begin to read while sitting, or lying on the ground. Move around all you want, but stay on the floor for as long as you can. You are already beginning the practice.

chapter one Yin Yoga Defined

Our goal in life is not to become perfect: our goal is to become whole.

Modern yoga has its roots deep in Eastern mysticism, has been fertilized by nineteenth-century gymnastics and wrestling, and has been shaped by Western sensibilities. Today, yoga as practiced in the West is totally unique: this yoga has never existed anywhere else before—today we practice Western Yoga for the benefits that Westerners desire. These benefits are considerable and will be explored in this investigation. If you have been doing yoga for a while now, you might be experiencing only half of the practice and just some of the benefits that are available to you. Yin Yoga is the other half.

Most forms of yoga today are dynamic, active practices designed to work only half of our body, the muscular half, the "yang" tissues. Yin Yoga allows us to work the other half, the deeper "yin" tissues of our ligaments, joints, deep fascial networks, and even our bones. All of our tissues are important and need to be exercised so that we can achieve optimal health and vitality.

Exercise our joints?! Isn't that dangerous? Yes and no. It depends on how we do it; we can exercise our joints safely if we do so intelligently. If done incorrectly, we can definitely hurt ourselves, but we can say that about any form of exercise.

Saying that Yin Yoga is the other half, that it works the deeper tissues of the body, is just the beginning of defining what Yin Yoga is all about. We need to look at the definitions of the underlying principles of yin and yoga to look at the intention behind engaging in a yoga practice, and to explore the benefits and methodologies used in a Yin Yoga practice.

There are many reasons for beginning a yoga practice; obtaining optimum physical health is just one. Many people are drawn to yoga to help reduce the effects of stress in their lives. Others wish to deepen their meditation practices or to simply become more present in their daily lives. As we will discover, yoga in general and Yin Yoga in particular provides physical, mental, emotional, and energetic benefits and, for some, spiritual. Which benefits you enjoy will depend greatly upon your intention when you practice.

How you practice is just as important as what you do in your practice. There is a yin aspect to life and a yang aspect. There is a yin way to practice yoga and a yang way that go beyond the actual movements and postures employed in a yoga session. Yin is yielding, allowing, and nourishing. Even within an active, sweaty yang practice we can adopt a yin sensitivity that will help us gain much more from our yoga practice. Even within an active yang lifestyle, we can adopt a yin awareness and acceptance that will help us gain contentment in our lives.

Yin Yoga can have the same goals and objectives as any other school of yoga. What we do will be different but *how* we do it will be the biggest difference. Why we do yoga really comes down to our own unique, particular intentions. Knowing the benefits of the Yin Yoga style will help you clarify intentions for your practice.

Some students initially find this style of yoga quite boring, passive, or soft, but they quickly discover that it can be quite challenging due to the long duration of the poses. Yin Yoga is simple, but simple does not mean easy. We can remain in the postures anywhere from one to twenty minutes! After you have experienced this, even just once, you will realize that you have been doing only half of the asana practice.

▷▷▷ **Please Note!** Yin Yoga as described here is *not* restorative yoga. If the tissues you are targeting for exercise are damaged in some way, please give yourself a chance to heal before resuming your regular practice.

Yin and Yang

Patterns define our lives. Look around you right now and you will notice the patterns surrounding you. Look up; you will see things that are high. Look down; you will see things that are low. Listen; you will hear things close by, and you will hear things far away. Bring your attention inward; you may feel the tip of your nose or the top of your head. Now you may be feeling the tips of your toes. Up, down ... near, far ... these are just some of the adjectives we can choose to describe the patterns of life, of existence. All patterns are formed by contrasts. The pattern on a chessboard is formed by the contrast of dark and light. The pattern of your life, when reflected upon, has displayed a contrast of good times and bad. For the Daoist, harmony and health are created when conditions arise where the contrasting aspects are in balance.

Balancing is not a static act. Imagine the typical depiction of weighing scales: two plates held by a common string suspended at a point halfway between them. When two equally weighted objects are placed upon the scales, there is a slight swaying motion, like a pendulum. If one side is too heavy, the scales tip and balance is lost. When both sides are equal, there is still a slight oscillation around the middle position. This rebalancing is the return to wholeness and health.

The ancient Chinese called this middle

YIN	YANG
Dark	Light
Cold	Hot
Passive	Active
Inside	Outside
Solid	Hollow
Slow	Rapid
Dim	Bright
Downward	Upward
Substance	Function
Water	Fire
Matter	Energy
Mysterious	Obvious
Female	Male
Moon	Sun
Night	Day
Earth	Heaven
Even	Odd
Dragon	Tiger
Plastic	Elastic

that we return to the Dao.[1] The Dao is the tranquility found in the center of all events, and the path leading to the center. The center is always there even if we are not always there to enjoy it. When we leave the center we take on aspects of yin or yang.

Yin and yang are relative terms: they describe the two facets of existence. Like two sides of one coin, yin cannot exist without yang, nor yang without yin. They complement each other. Since existence is never static, what is yin and what is yang are always in flux, always changing.

The ancient Chinese observed that everything has yin or yang attributes. The terms existed in Confucianism and in the earliest Daoist writings. The yin character refers to the shady side of a hill or stream. Yang refers to the sunny side. Shade cannot exist without light, and light can only be light when contrasted to darkness. And so we see how, even in the earliest uses of these terms, patterns are observed.

There is no absolute yin or absolute yang. A context is always required: in the context of light, darkness and brightness define yin and yang. In a number of other contexts, yin describes what is relatively denser, heavier, lower, more hidden, more yielding, more feminine, more mysterious, and more passive. Yang describes the opposite conditions: what is less dense, lighter, higher, more obvious or superficial, more masculine, and more dynamic. The table shows a more complete list of comparisons. There is no limit to the relative contexts in which yin and yang can be applied.

Yin Contains Yang

Look again at the symbol for yin and yang at the beginning of this section. Do you see the white dot within the dark paisley swirl? Even within the darkness of yin, there is a lightness of yang and vice versa. In the context of temperature we say that hotter is yang and cooler is yin; but hot water is yin compared to boiling water, which is yang. In the other direction, cold water is yang compared to ice, which is yin.

In our yoga practice there are very active asana workouts, which we may call yang, but even within these yang practices we can find yin aspects; watching our breath mindfully while we flow through a vigorous vinyasa[2] is just one example.

Yin Becomes Yang

Just as we detect yin elements within the yang aspects, we can also notice how yin becomes yang, and yang can transform into yin. These transformations may be slow and subtle, or they may be devastatingly quick. The seasons roll slowly by, changing imperceptibly. The yang of spring and summer transforms day by day into the yin of fall and winter. It is not possible to pick the exact moment at which one season becomes another, astronomical observations notwithstanding. But the transformation may also come quickly: the eye of a hurricane quickly brings calm, and just as quickly the eye moves on and the other half of the storm strikes.

In our own life we often experience both the slow and quick transformations of yin into yang and yang into yin. We wake up in the morning; yin becomes yang. Sometimes our awakening is slow, leisurely; this is a slow transformation. Sometimes we wake with a start and jump out of bed, perhaps because we overslept. When we work long hours for many weeks or months in a row (a very yang lifestyle), our body may seek balance by suddenly making us too sick to work (a very yin lifestyle), or it may gift us with a severe migraine to slow us down. Yang is quickly transformed into yin.

Yin Controls Yang

In this last example, we can see that if we stay too long in an unbalanced situation, the universe acts to restore balance. It throws us to the other side: our health may suffer and our lives may change. If we do not heed the need for balancing yin and yang, this transition can be devastating. A heart attack could be the balancing force applied to us. These imbalances are often referred to as an excess or a deficiency. We can have an excess or a deficiency of either yin or yang. The cure is to apply the opposite energy to control the imbalance.

In the Eastern world of the yogis[3] of India and the alchemical Daoists of China, the need for balance is well known and understood.[4] In the West, while we do not use the terms yin and yang, the need to pay attention and balance our opposing natures has been realized by many astute observers of our psychological landscape. Carl Jung recognized his dark side, which he termed "the shadow," and discovered that if left unattended, these dark, repressed energies will wreak havoc in one's life. The oppositions within create a dynamic tension that can lead to destruction or amazing creativity. For Jung, the way to work with these opposing energies is to integrate them, or individuate[5]. He, and his followers after him, developed many tools to do this integration. Shadow work can include active imagining or creating rituals that honor both energies within us.

SPIRITUAL	PRACTICAL
Losing	Winning
Outgo	Income
Fasting	Eating
Passivity	Action
Giving	Earning
Poverty	Possession
Repose	Activity
Celibacy	Sex
Observation	Decisiveness
Obedience	Freedom
Duty	Choice
Ecstasy	Sobriety
Vision	Focus
Less is more	More is better

Notice the differences and the similarities between the earlier table of yin and yang characteristics with the table on the previous page, taken from Robert Johnson's[6] book *Owning Your Own Shadow*. Here, Johnson shows the many opposing values we are subjected to in Western cultures:[7] one set our religious or spiritual beliefs require of us, and the other set is what we need to survive and thrive in our secular life, the business world. Note the yin-like qualities and the opposing yang-like energies. How we reconcile the opposing energies of Sunday morning versus the rest of the week will lead either to a breakdown or a breakthrough; a revelation—which is only possible if we do the work required, if we do our yoga whether with Western or Eastern techniques.

In the West, true understanding of yin and yang is uncommon. We don't think in these terms; our lifestyles rarely reflect the need for balance. We seek it only when the universe forces us to pay attention, when we suffer the breakdown that avoiding our dark side creates. Only then do we seek help to regain balance. Only when we become exhausted or sick do we take time off. Only when we injure our bodies do we slow down and look for gentler ways to exercise. We can be yang-like for only so long before crashing. We can be yin-like for only so long before stagnating. We need balance in all things.

Yin Tissues and Yang Tissues

As mentioned, yin and yang are relative terms and need a context to be appropriately applied. They can be used as adjectives, although they are often used as nouns. Within our bodies, if we use the context of position or density, the yang tissues can be seen as our muscles, blood, and skin compared to the yin tissues of ligaments, bones, and joints. The contexts of flexibility or heat could also be used: muscles are elastic, but bones are plastic.[8] Muscles love to get warm, while ligaments generally remain cool.

Yang styles of yoga generally target the muscles and employ rhythmic, repetitive movements to stress the fibers and cells of the muscles. Being elastic and moist, the muscles appreciate this form of exercise and respond well to it. Yin tissues, however, being dryer and much less elastic, could be damaged if they were stressed in this way. Instead, our more plastic tissues appreciate and require gentler pressures, applied for longer periods of time, in order to be stimulated to grow stronger. This is why orthodontic braces must be worn for a long time with a reasonable (but not always comfortable) amount of pressure, in order to reshape the bones of the jaw.

Our joints can be seen simply as spaces between the bones where movement is possible. Stabilizing the joint are ligaments, muscles, and tendons, which bind the bones together. Generally, one of the muscles' jobs is to protect the joint; if there is too much stress on the joint, the muscle will tear first, then the ligaments, and then finally the joint itself may become damaged. In this regard, yang yoga is designed to *not* stress the joint. This is why there is so much care taken to align the body and engage the muscles correctly before coming into asanas in the yang practice. However, Yin Yoga is specifically designed to exercise the ligaments and to regain space and strength in the joints.

An example can help explain the different roles of the muscles and ligaments. Place your right index finger in your left hand. Extend the finger and tighten the muscles and, with your left hand, try to bend the finger upwards. Notice that there is virtually no movement. The muscles' job is to bind the bones together and limit the range of motion allowed in the joint. Now relax the finger completely. Shake it out for a moment. Now, keeping the muscles passive, try to push the finger upwards. Notice the difference? The relaxed finger can move 90 degrees or more. When the muscles are relaxed the stress is moved to the ligaments binding the joint.

Stability and Mobility

Remember the white dot within the paisley swirl of the yin and yang symbol? Within yang there is yin and vice versa; this also applies to our tissues. Consider the muscle, which we just described as a yang tissue. Even here we will find yin within yang: 30 percent of what we call our muscle is actually fascia. As we will discover, it is the fascia within our muscles that govern the muscles' range of movement while it is our muscle cells that govern their strength. Yang yoga is great at developing the yang attribute of strength within our muscles but, surprisingly perhaps, it is the yin part of our practice, the holding of the pose, that provides length.

Within our yin tissues, we also find yang elements. In our fascia and ligaments, which are predominantly yin-like, there are contracting fibers, just like within our muscles. We also find elastic fibers called elastin within our yin tissues. So there is yang within yin here, too: our connective tissues can contract and shorten.

Physiologically, through our yoga practice, we build stability and mobility. If we look at the arc of aging, which everyone follows albeit at faster or slower rates, we begin life completely yang-like: we have the ultimate mobility that we will ever have, but we have no stability. Newborn babies have to be handled carefully because they have no internal stability. Now we start to stiffen, to become more yin-like. We gain stability as we age. When we are youngsters, we don't need to work on gaining more mobility because we are already so yang-like: we need to work on our muscles and gaining strength. This is a yang time of life so we need yang forms of exercise.[9] Somewhere around our mid-twenties to mid-thirties we reach the optimal balance between yin and yang, between mobility and stability. But the arc of aging must be followed: we continue to become more yin-like as we age, until eventually we end up completely rigid, as rigor mortis sets into our dead bodies. As we get older, as we get more yin-like, we need a yin form of exercise to keep us mobile.

The Theory of Exercise

All forms of exercise share two features in common:
   ▷ first we must stress the tissues,
   ▷ then we must let the tissues rest.

Yang tissues do better when stressed in a yang manner and yin tissues do better when stressed in a yin way. Stress has many negative connotations in our culture because we forget the "rest" part of this equation. But to have no, or little, stress in our life is just as damaging as having too much stress. We need to stress the body, and we need to rest it. There is a yin/yang balance here that leads to health. Too much of anything is not healthy.

Yang exercise targets the yang tissues: the muscles. Muscles love to be rhythmically and repetitively moved. Any static holds are brief[10]. The muscles are elastic and can take this type of exercise. However, to apply yang exercise to yin tissues could damage them. Yin tissues, being more plastic, require gentler but long-held stresses. Imagine bending a credit card back and forth one hundred and eight times every morning, over and over again. It wouldn't take many mornings of this for it to snap in half. The credit card is plastic, just as our ligaments are. To rhythmically bend ligaments over and over again, as some students do when doing drop back from standing into the Wheel or moving from Up-dog to Down-dog, can, over time, damage the ligaments, just like the credit card was damaged. The warning here is ... **do not apply yang exercise techniques to yin tissues!**

Applying a yin exercise to yang tissues could also be damaging. Holding a muscle in a contracted state for a long period of time is called "tetany"[11] and may damage it.

Is it better to tighten muscles (yang) or relax them (yin)? That depends on your intention. We tighten our muscles to protect our joints. We relax our muscles so we can exercise our joints. What is your intention in the pose you are doing?

Many health care professionals shudder at the thought of exercising joints; they have the mistaken view that all exercise is yang exercise. Despite this concern it is possible to exercise ligaments, bones, and joints in a yin way. In fact, it is necessary.

However, because they are yin tissues we must exercise them in a yin way. And please remember the important second part of this equation—we must rest![12] There is a lot of research proving the importance of stress and rest beyond just developing strength physically, but it is beyond the scope of this journey to go into it further.[13]

Stretch Versus Stress

We need to define a couple of terms that are used rather loosely by many yoga teachers: stress and stretch. These are not synonyms. Technically, stress is the tension that we place upon our tissues, while stretch is the elongation that results from the stress. We often say we are stretching our muscles, but to be more precise, what we are doing is applying a stress to our muscles that results in a stretch. A stretch, however, does not always accompany a stress, so they are not the same thing. For example, in isometric exercises we stress the muscles, but there is no change in the length of the muscles.

We can stress ligaments too, especially in Yin Yoga, but because the ligaments are more plastic and less elastic than muscles, that stress is less likely to result in a stretch. There may be some small stretch to a ligament; however, generally the tendons and ligaments should not stretch more than 4–10 percent or we risk damaging them.[14] We are *not* trying to stretch our ligaments or joint capsules with Yin Yoga. We *are* trying to stress them. Over time, the tissues may become longer, thicker, and stronger, but in any one Yin Yoga session, we are not trying to lengthen these particular tissues. Said another way, in Yin Yoga, the key is the stress not the stretch.

When we use the term *stretch* in this book, we will either refer to a lengthening of the tissues (for example, we will stretch a muscle to make it longer) or we will use it to indicate that the intention of the applied stress is to lengthen the tissues, even if no lengthening actually occurs. If we are not intending to lengthen the tissues, which is mostly the case in Yin Yoga, we will not use the term *stretch*, but will stick to the term *stress*.

Original Yin

A seal discovered during the excavation of Mohenjo-Daro, one of the largest cities of the ancient Harappan civilization, which flourished over 4,000 years ago, depicts a yogi sitting in a meditative posture—and a Yin Yoga posture at that.

Hatha Yoga, the most common form of yoga practiced today in the West, is a physical practice. The intention of Hatha Yoga, which blossomed around the tenth century C.E., was to prepare the body for the more advanced yoga practices of meditation and insight. Hatha Yoga arose out of the earlier Tantra Yoga style, which in turn drew from the Classical Yoga of around 2,000 years ago.

There has never been one yoga from which all other yogas have evolved. There is no yoga-tree that one can create to show the inter-relationships between all the various forms and expressions of yoga over the millennia. Rather, we would need to draw a forest of yoga trees to really understand yoga's full and varied history. We do know that Hatha Yoga as a specific practice is not itself thousands of years old, but Hatha Yoga does have roots that go back that far. It is known that ancient yogas from many lineages incorporated some basic physical practices, such as sitting in meditation, as shown in the seal mentioned above.

Sitting for long periods of time is a yin form of exercise. If you have ever tried to sit for even one hour at a time, you know this is not easy. To sit for hours upon hours every day requires special training of the body and the mind; the back muscles need to be strong, the posture needs to be correct, the hips need to be open, and the mind needs to be focused. While there are no extant texts from 2,000 years ago or earlier that describe how these ancient meditators prepared their bodies for these exertions, we can safely assume that they did prepare their bodies in some way. One of the best ways to prepare you for a specific yoga pose is to do that specific pose! One way to best prepare ourselves to sit, is to sit. Sitting, quietly for a long period of time, is a yin practice. We can speculate that most, if not all, of the earliest asana practices were yin-like in nature. However, it did not stay that way.

There are just a few texts that have survived the centuries that describe the way Hatha Yoga was taught in the tenth to eighteenth centuries: the Hatha Yoga Pradipika, the Gheranda Samhita, the Shiva Samhita, and a few others. However, none of these ancient texts were meant to be read alone. They all required the guidance of a guru to ensure understanding.

The books were used more like notes—shorthand reminders of the real teaching. Much of the real knowledge was deliberately kept hidden; only when the teacher felt the student was ready was the knowledge revealed. We cannot tell simply from reading these old texts how the physical practice of yoga was performed. What we can say, as mentioned earlier, is that the purpose of the physical practice was to prepare the student for the deeper practices of meditation.

In the earliest spiritual books of India, the Vedas, yoga is not described as a path to liberation, and asana practice is not described at all. Rather, *yoga*, among its many other meanings, meant discipline, and the closest word to *asana* was *asundi*, which described a block upon which one sat in order to meditate. By the time the Yoga Sutra was compiled,[15] yoga was defined as a psycho-spiritual practice aimed at ultimate liberation. Asana, however, was still a very minor aspect of the practice. The Yoga Sutra mentions asana only twice[16] in all one hundred and ninety-six aphorisms. And all that is said about asana is that it should be *sthira* and *sukham*: steady and comfortable. These are very much yin qualities, compared to the style of asana we see performed today in yoga classes. When we are still and the mind undistracted by bodily sensation, meditation can arise.

The point of yoga practices is to enter into a meditative state from which realization or liberation may arise. Different schools of yoga have different techniques for achieving this. Some even claim that one cannot become liberated while in the body. The goal in these early dualistic schools is to get out of the body as fast as possible, but this must be done in the right way. Other schools rejected that approach and suggested, since we can only meditate and practice yoga while in the body, we must treat the body well. The body must be healthy. The focus of the Hatha Yoga schools was to build a strong, healthy body that would allow the yogi to meditate for many hours each day. In Hatha Yoga, the practice of asana began to take on a new, broader importance. However, the ultimate goal was still to be able to sit comfortably and steadily for hours.

The Hatha Yoga Pradipika was written around 1350 C.E. by Swami Swatmarama.[17] It is almost twice as long as the Yoga Sutra and has generated a lot of commentary since its writing. It is one of the oldest extant documents we have describing Hatha Yoga. Compared to today's practices, however, it too has very little asana practice in it. There are only fifteen asanas listed, and of these, eight are seated postures.[18] These are quite yin-like in their nature; however, many of the other postures are definitely yang-like. The peacock (*mayurasana*) is prescribed, and if you have seen this posture performed, there is nothing relaxing or yin-like about it. We are told that one of the fifteen postures is supreme; once one has mastered *siddhasana*, all the other postures are useless.[19] Siddhasana is a simple, yin-like seated posture.

The Hatha Yoga Pradipika claims that Lord Shiva taught the Hatha Yoga sage Matsyendra eighty-four asanas.[20] Other myths claim there are eighty-four thousand or even eight hundred and forty thousand asanas. Regardless, only fifteen are listed in the Pradipika. And of asanas it is said that these should be practiced to gain steady posture, health, and lightness of the body.[21] Not mentioned in any of the Hatha texts is how long one should hold the pose. This is where the guru's guidance is necessary. However, one can assume that the seated postures were meant to be held a long time while the more vigorous poses like the peacock were held for briefer periods. It is in the seated postures that the *vayus* (the winds or the breath) become trained through *pranayama*. The Lotus Pose (*padmasana*) is the prescribed pose for conducting pranayama.[22]

As time went on, later texts expanded the number of asanas explained. The Gheranda Samhita, written perhaps in the late 1600s,[23] a few hundred years after the Pradipika, describes thirty-two asanas, of which one-third could be said to be yin-like and the others more yang-like. A trend had begun: more yang asanas than yin asanas. A few decades later, the Shiva Samhita listed eighty-four asanas. By the time of the British Raj, when England began to colonize Indian culture and change the school system, asanas were beginning to become blended with forms from the gymnasiums. Wrestling, gymnastics, and other exercises were cross-fertilizing the asana practice. By the end of the nineteenth century there were thousands of asanas. Krishnamacharya[24] said he knew around three thousand postures but that his guru, Ramamohan Brahmachari, knew eight thousand. The era of yang yoga was upon us.

This gradual, and then sudden, evolution of asana practice moved it away from the original yin style of holding seated poses for a long time as a preparation for the deeper practice of meditation to the more active yang style of building strength and health. It is not that the more yin-like poses disappeared: B.K.S. Iyengar, in his *Light on Yoga*, suggests that the pose Supta Virasana[25] should be held for ten to fifteen minutes. That is Yin Yoga, he just never used that terminology.[26] Theos Bernard, a very popular Hatha Yoga teacher in the mid-twentieth century, also recommended long holds of various postures. The problem arose that, despite yin-like poses remaining in the lexicon of asanas, they were marginalized in favor of the more yang-like postures. One is not better than the other; they are simply different. To sit for long periods of time in deep, undisturbed meditation requires a body that is open and strong. This opening, especially in the hips and lower back, is developed through a dedicated yin practice. However, there is certainly nothing wrong with working the heart and making our muscles longer and stronger, too.

The original styles of physical yoga were very yin-like in nature. Over the past two hundred years the style has changed to be more yang-like. As in all things in life, harmony comes through balance. By combining both styles, progress in practice is more assured. But, why do we call this "Yin" yoga? *Yin* is not an Indian term, it is a Chinese word. Where did this crossover come from? Let's look at the parallel development of physical yoga from a Chinese, or Daoist, perspective.

Daoist Yoga

Ten thousand years ago throughout all cultures, shamans blazed the spiritual paths. In India the shamanic traditions evolved into the yogic practices and philosophies we have been investigating. But this evolution was not confined to the valleys of the Indus, Saraswati (now gone), and Ganges rivers. In Europe (especially in Greece), the Middle East, and China, the same discoveries were being made. Over centuries, despite the distance and difficulty of travel, knowledge filtered out and was shared between cultures. It is not surprising that we find similar concepts discussed in the spiritual practices and philosophies of each region. However, the models and metaphors were modified to fit the local cultural landscape.

The concept of spirit (breath) in the European world had its counterpart in prana (breath) in India. In China the same energy was known as *Chi*. Chi is just one of several concepts central to Chinese medical practices. These concepts evolved out of native spiritual practices grouped together under the name Daoism.[27]

There are many forms of Daoism and many ways to practice the teachings. The Dao is sometimes personalized as a god, but most often it is impersonalized as a benevolent but disinterested power: the way of the universe. Live in harmony with the way and you will benefit. Struggle against the way things are and you will suffer.

Most Westerners know of the Dao through the book by Lao-tzu called the *Dao De Ching: The Way of Virtue.*[28] In the *Dao De Ching* we are taught that the Dao is the source of everything. It is nameless because whenever you try to capture the essence of the universe in a concept, you miss the totality of what you are trying to name. The Dao is infinite and inexhaustible. Only the Dao is unchanging and unchangeable.

Since everything is part of the Dao, it follows that the earth, sky, rivers, mountains, stars, and humans are also part of the Dao. Man is not outside of all this but part of it.[29] In the *Dao De Ching* the message is: Get involved! Help, but help in a non-intrusive way. When finished, retire. Yang is acting. Yin is retiring. The Dao is the balance between the two.

In the Daoism of Lao-tzu, the sage is one who cultivates life. The sage learns physical techniques to do this: he regulates his breath, he hones his body, he garners health, and he manages his internal energies including the important sexual energy. Along with the physical techniques, the sage also follows ethical principles and regulates his own mind through meditation. Diet is also an important part of building and maintaining health. Through all these practices, the sage seeks to change his body and mind to recover youth and vitality and live in peace.

The Five Major Systems

There are five main systems in Daoism. These are sometimes contradictory and confusing, especially to people of different cultures. Many of the practices of one system are used in the other systems. Thus, the lines between these systems are not fixed and final. The five systems are:

1. **Magical Daoism**: the oldest form of Daoism still practiced today. In this practice, the powers of the elements of nature and spirits are invoked and channeled through the practitioner to gain health, wealth, and progeny.

2. **Divinational Daoism**: based on understanding the way of the universe and seeing the great patterns of life. Knowing how the universe works allows us to live in harmony with those universal forces. As in heaven, so on earth. Divinational Daoism utilizes the study of the stars and patterns found on earth to help us live harmoniously. The *I-Ching* (the book of changes) is a divinational book.

3. **Ceremonial Daoism**: Daoism was originally a spiritual practice. Unlike yoga, which remained a personal spiritual practice, this branch of Daoism evolved into a religion.

4. **Action and Karma Daoism**: Proper action leads to accumulating merit. Following the introduction of Buddhism into China, ethics took on a greater role in spiritual practice. But it did not start there; Confucius also taught the value of proper behaviour and morality. Good deeds result in rewards, both in this life and the next.

5. **Internal Alchemy Daoism**: Immortality is the goal of this practice. The seeker works to change his mind and body to achieve health and longevity. It was in this practice that Chi became recognized as the key to health and long life. Chi is gathered, nurtured, and circulated through very strict practices. Incorrect practice is dangerous, and this path of Daoism required an expert teacher. It is mostly from this system that Chinese medicine evolved.

While an investigation of all these forms of Daoism is beyond the scope of this book, we can look in more detail at the really interesting branch—Alchemical Daoism. [30]

Alchemical Daoism

The Indian yogis were seeking spiritual immortality: liberation from the endless cycles of death and rebirth. The Daoist yogis, who practiced alchemical Daoism, were seeking physical immortality: they simply wanted to live forever in this body. The form of alchemy we are talking about is not the transformation of base materials to gold, but the transformation of the normal body to a perfect body. Changing lead to gold is a metaphor for the real goal. There was a period where external alchemy was tried, which involved a lot of poisonous substances like mercury, but after hundreds of years of simply poisoning the seeker to death, this form of alchemy was dropped in favor of an internal method—to change from within.

To become physically immortal, one needed to become really healthy, and that required a lot of dedication and hard work. It could be done! Or at least, it was known that a few amazing individuals had achieved immortality, but these Daoist immortals were not easy to find and we can assume they are mythological beings, not living humans whom we can email and ask how they did it. And, to be sure, there are many who believe that the real immortality that alchemical Daoists seek is spiritual immortality, once this mortal coil has been shed. In either case, spiritual immortality or physical immortality, the practice of the internal alchemical Daoists is every bit as challenging as the Indian yoga practices.

The first priority of an internal alchemist is to conserve his energies. When we are born, we are given a certain amount of three main kinds of energy: generative energy (called *Jing*), which feeds our sexual desires, vital energy (the commonly known Chi energy), and spirit energy (called *Shen*). While these energies are filling us up as we grow in our mother's womb, the mind and the body are already starting to separate. When we are born, out of our ignorance we begin to dissipate our three main energies. We lose our generative energy any time we even think about sex. Our Chi leaks out through our emotions, and our Shen is lost when our thoughts flow. These leakages are what weaken us, cause illness, and lead ultimately to our death.[31] Through alchemical practice, through internal transformation, our original stores of energy can be rebuilt and we can regain health and longevity.

Alchemical Daoism focuses on the stimulation and balancing of energy in both its yin and yang aspects. The yin energy is the dragon: the yang energy is the tiger. To unify yin and yang we must remove all blockages that exist throughout the body so that these energies can unite in the three cauldrons, called the tan-t'iens.[32] The process to stimulate these energies involves our breath. Fast breathing will direct yang fire to the middle and upper cauldrons, while slower and softer breathing will stimulate yin energy to incubate our internal energies.

Transformation also involves physical and mental exercises to change our skeletal structures and our mental formations. Before working on the mental changes, one must master the physical changes. Tools here include a host of exercises designed to hone the body: tendon-changing practices, massage, martial arts, and the more widely known t'ai chi ch'uan and ch'i-kung practices. Once this basic training is successful, the alchemist moves on to transform his internal energy. Refining and transforming generative energy, which is stored in the kidneys, into vital energy involves work in the abdomen area, physically, as well as mental practices to minimize sexual desires. Care now must be taken not to dissipate our vital energy through negative emotions, such as anger, fear, frustration, or sadness. Now the alchemist is ready for the final stage: transforming vital energy into spirit energy. For this, meditation is required. The mind must become empty of thoughts, and all signs of duality extinguished. There is no longer a subject and an object: no thinker and no thought.

When the alchemist is sufficiently advanced, he is ready to begin to circulate his energy through a practice known as the microcosmic orbit.[33] He will not be successful if he has not first cleared out all the blockages to the flow of energy or if his mind or senses are stimulated. In the 1930s, Richard Wilhelm[34] described the benefit of the circling of light in his translation of *The Secret of the Golden Flower, a Chinese Book of Life*. This ancient text was transmitted orally for centuries before being written down in the eighth century. Wilhelm, a friend of Carl Jung's, wrote:

> If the life forces flow downward, that is, without let or hindrance into the outer world, the anima is victorious over the animus; no "spirit body" or "Golden Flower" is developed, and, at death, the ego is lost. If the life forces are led through the "backward-flowing" process, that is, conserved, and made to "rise" instead of allowed to dissipate, the animus has been victorious, and the ego persists after death. It is then possessed of shen, the revealing spirit. A man who holds to the way of conservation all through life may reach the stage of the "Golden Flower," which then frees the ego from the conflict of the opposites, and it again becomes part of Tao, the undivided, Great One.

Success at last! Immortality is achieved through the inner alchemical practice of changing the body, managing energy, and meditations. Along the way many herbs and other dietary rules are followed. Lifestyle changes are also required. This is not an easy path.

Cultivating the Body

Tendon-changing? What the heck is that? How do we change our tendons and why is that so important? Good questions. The Daoists use terms that sound familiar to our Western ears, but they don't quite mean the same thing as what we think. For example, the word *organs*, to our Western mind refers to physically differentiated tissues that perform specific functions, located in one specific area of the body. To the Daoist, however, *Organs*[35] refers to the physical organs as we know and love them in the West, but also to an Organ function dispersed throughout the body. Similarly Blood, to our Daoist friends, doesn't just flow through our veins, it flows through our meridians and nourishes our tendons. Tendons are more than what we think of in our Western viewpoint, which are simply the connective tissues that join a muscle to a bone. In Daoism, Tendons[36] include ligaments and muscles, fascia and nerves, as well as other soft body tissues.

Tendon-changing practices are ones that target a wide range of tissues and involve stressing, strengthening, and massaging these tissues. Of interest to our exploration is the fact that tendon-changing deliberately targets not just the muscles, but also the joints and ligaments; the intention is to regain our natural, dynamic state, our original or optimal ranges of motions. The Daoist practices for cultivating the body include both yin and yang forms of exercises, just as the original Hatha Yoga practices did.

Bone exercises include a technique called "Marrow-washing." Fortunately we don't actually extract our bone marrow and clean it before sucking it back in. This is Marrow, not marrow. Marrow washing incorporates slow, smooth pressure applied to our joints and the bones. This is a yin-like way to stress the bones and joints; there is a more yang-like way, which involves hitting and grinding the bones, but that technique is quite esoteric.

Breath work is also very important in order to really cultivate the body. It includes deep abdominal breathing, natural and unforced, breathing through the mouth, through the nose, through both mouth and nose, through the perineum, and several other more esoteric practices. Tortoise breathing is notable: because tortoises live so long, they must be doing something right. They breathe very lightly when they are huddled inside their shells. In fact, they barely breathe at all.[37]

No doubt you are familiar already with some of the classical exercises performed in Daoism called t'ai chi ch'uan and ch'i-kung. These practices look like slow-motion calisthenics, but really they are designed to move energy internally. They combine stretching, breathing, and meditation. They can be performed while sitting, standing, and even walking. They can also be performed when sleeping, but this is not the shavasana that we all enjoy at the end of our Hatha Yoga practice. If our tendons are healthy and soft, if our energy channels are open, then these practices will facilitate the flow of inner energy.

The earliest forms of Daoist exercises were developed after carefully observing animals in nature. Animals all move naturally, spontaneously, and in harmony with the Dao.[38] If we copy their movements, we can gain the same connection to the Dao that they have. Five special animals were valued highly for their movements: the tiger and the dragon, who epitomize yang and yin, the crane, leopard, and snake. As Eva Wong says:[39]

The tiger is valued for its strong bones, the leopard for its dynamic tendons, the dragon for its ability in stretching the spine, the snake for its flexibility in moving the spine, and the crane for its capacity to store internal energy.

Of course, these were not the only animals that were being watched closely. Another fascinating creature was the monkey.

Modern Yinsters

Around the turn of the nineteenth century, a prisoner who was sentenced to eight years in solitary confinement for killing a man spent his time studying the monkeys he could see from his cell.[40] He studied their movements for years and combined them with a form of martial arts that he had learned as a child. Upon his release from prison, he taught his new form of martial arts, called Tai Shing Men (Monkey Kung-fu).[41] His teaching eventually found its way to Hong Kong, where a student named Cho Chat Ling learned this style of practice from his uncle. In the 1970s Cho Chat Ling moved to California.

Paulie Zink

While flipping through TV channels in 1987, Paul Grilley noticed someone who really caught his eye: the guy being interviewed on this community cable station was Paulie Zink. Paul had been teaching yoga since 1980 and was used to seeing flexible bodies, but he had never seen anyone as flexible and graceful in his movements as Paulie.[42] Paul resolved to meet him, and through the community TV station, located him. Paulie was teaching Monkey Kung-fu from his garage, where he earned a living as a mechanic. It was in this garage that Paulie gave Paul his first lesson in Daoist Yoga.[43] What really caught Paul's eye was the yin aspect of Daoist Yoga, the long-held poses that Paulie would enjoy, although his students would use the term "endure." Paul joined the small group of students studying with Paulie and for the next year took weekly lessons with him.

After Cho Chat Ling relocated to the US, he began to search for someone to whom he could pass on the training that his uncle had taught him. Passing on the training is the obligation of every student: once a master has completed training you, your job is to find and train the next generation of students. Cho Chat Ling found his protégé in Paulie. Paulie had been studying martial arts since his teenage years, but when he met Master Cho during his college years, he dedicated himself to this new teaching. Master Cho would come to Paulie's home and teach him for six to eight hours every day for seven years! Half of the training was Daoist Yoga and the other half was martial arts. After the seventh year, Master Cho's visits were less frequent, and by the tenth year, he declared Paulie his successor. Master Cho eventually returned to Asia, leaving Paulie to continue to spread the knowledge. At no time did Master Cho charge for his teaching.

Paulie did share what he learned, and he shared it in a similar manner to the way he was taught. The classes he offered were long, often starting at 8 p.m. and lasting until 1 or 2 in the morning.

The style of teaching offered by Cho Chat Ling, and then by Paulie, was not traditional: they added their own personalities to it. No longer was the training rigid; now it was art, celestial art, unobtainable in a weekend workshop but possible within a long-term intimate relationship with a teacher. Master Cho taught Paulie Daoist alchemical theory but Paulie's innate flexibility allowed him to take this even further. It was Paulie who discovered the deep, juicy benefits of marinating in one position for a long, long time. Paulie eventually programmed his martial arts training into a "now we do some yoga" phase and then the martial arts phase. Sometimes Paulie would refer to the yoga as "the internal practice" or as "chi kung."

Paulie's yoga was nothing like any Indian yoga teacher would have taught. There were a few poses that would have been familiar to Indian yogis, such as the splits (Hanumanasana and Upavistakonasana) and other seated folding poses, held for long periods, but Paulie also included the movements of the five elements. This was his only formal meditation teaching: move like each element. The elementary movements would be combined into the birthing cycles and the controlling cycles. Paulie would also incorporate animal movements: the bear, the lizard and, of course, the monkey were just a few. In essence, Paulie's teaching included both yin and yang elements, which comprised his full expression of Daoist Yoga.

He never had a large group of students and charged virtually nothing for his time, but Paulie grew discouraged by the quality of the students seeking his knowledge. Most students, coming from a martial arts background, were only interested in learning the secret ways to hurt and even kill their enemies. Paulie never wanted to share that information and he eventually moved to a bucolic lifestyle on a ranch outside of Billings, Montana. After trying to teach yoga at a small studio in Billings, Paulie withdrew entirely from teaching. Fortunately, this retirement was short-lived. In recent years, Paulie has returned to share his vast knowledge.

Paulie's seminars and workshops are quite different from the Yin Yoga practice as taught by Paul Grilley and Sarah Powers; Paulie continues to offer the full range of Daoist Yoga, including explorations of the five elements in movement and postures. Attending one of Paulie's workshops is just the first step in understanding the whole body of knowledge that he inherited and augmented. You can read more about him on his website.[44]

Paul Grilley

Years before Paul Grilley discovered Paulie Zink, he became inspired to investigate yoga after reading Yogananada's *Autobiography of a Yogi* in 1979. Paul was living in Montana where he was studying anatomy under Dr. Garry Parker. Paul decided to move to Los Angeles and continued studying anatomy at UCLA. While there, Paul also began his studies of yoga, and began teaching as well, eventually even managing a studio. Paul's main asana practices at this time were very yang: Ashtanga and Bikram's.

Yoga and anatomy are intimately linked, and Paul's investigations in these two fields informed each other greatly. Outside of Paul's fame as a popularizer of Yin Yoga, he has also contributed greatly to the understanding of how our unique anatomical structure ultimately affects our range of motion: in essence, not everyone can do every yoga pose, and for some people, to attempt to try to obtain an aesthetically pleasing posture may seriously injure their body.[45]

Once Paul had been introduced to the yin side of yoga through Paulie, he began to incorporate this philosophy into his own teaching. Paul created classes, which he originally called Daoist Yoga in deference to the name Paulie used for the practice, that encompassed only the yin aspects: long-held, still postures.

In 1990 Paul met Dr. Hiroshi Motoyama of Japan.[46] Dr. Motoyama has Ph.D. degrees in philosophy and psychology and is a yogic adept; more than that, he has studied Traditional Chinese Medicine and is a highly respected Shinto priest. Early in his life Motoyama was also taken under the wing of his mother's teacher, who adopted the young Motoyama.[47] Dr. Motoyama's ability to move freely between the worlds of the spirit and of the physical allowed him to investigate his own abilities using the rigors of Western science and medicine. With the aim of making the subtle measurable, he created instruments that he and others have learned to use to verify and quantify the flow of energy through the subtle body.

To further his research and spread his findings, Dr. Motoyama created institutes both in Japan and in the US.[48] Paul was inspired by what Dr. Motoyama revealed and travelled with him to Japan to learn more.

What Paul learned explained why our yoga practice was so valuable energetically. From his anatomy training, Paul had pieced together many of the important physiological benefits of yoga in general and Yin Yoga in particular. Now he was beginning to understand the basis of the energetic benefits we also receive from our yoga practice. Dr. Motoyama's theory of the meridians (the way our body's physical and energetic structures are connected through the chakra system) and his scientific experiments demonstrated the effect on our whole body from yoga.

Paul combined the knowledge he had been given on anatomy, Daoist Yoga, and the meridian theory, and this became the core of his Yin Yoga teachings—which resonated with many people who recognized the benefits of the practice and related to Paul's model of the body/mind/soul.

From 1998 to 2000 Paul took a sabbatical and relocated to Santa Fe, where he earned a master's degree from St. John's College in the study of the Great Books of the Western World. More and more, Paul's teaching gravitated to the yin side. He would never completely give up the yang styles of yoga—after all, we do need balance in life. To share more broadly what he had learned from Paulie and Dr. Motoyama, in 2001 Paul decided to self-publish a manual called *Taoist Yoga*. This later became his book, *Yin Yoga*. It continues to be in demand and has been reprinted many times.

Along with his wife, Suzee, Paul travels the world leading workshops and trainings, not just on Yin Yoga but on anatomy and the subtle, energetic body. Paul has created several fascinating videos demonstrating how our unique anatomy affects our yoga practice. One of the most interesting pages on his website shows many human bones that Paul has selected to demonstrate the range of variation we have in our bodies and in our ultimate ranges of motions.[49]

Sarah Powers

One of the many students who loved Paul's teaching of Daoist Yoga was Sarah Powers. She was also a teacher at the same studio Paul taught at and would often come to his class after teaching her own. When Paul moved away, they lost contact, but fortunately, only for a little while.

Sarah Powers' journey into the world of yoga was unplanned. Her initial goal was to learn how her mind worked. She was earning a master's degree in psychology when the detour that was to consume her occurred: she chose to study a topic based upon a book that had been lying around her home for many years. It was a book on yoga; Sarah fell in love.

Fortunately, she was already married at the time this new direction appeared in her life. Supported by her husband, Ty, she was able to delve deeply into the practice of yoga. She took teacher-training courses and began teaching in Malibu. Her practice gravitated to the yang styles, but at that time she had no awareness that yoga could be yin or yang.

One day, after a lovely and sweaty Ashtanga class, Sarah tried a Daoist Yoga class Paul Grilley was teaching. That was her first taste of yin, and it was delicious. Sarah loved sinking deeply into the poses. However, at that time Paul's classes were mostly conducted in silence; he didn't explain the various and deep benefits that Yin Yoga has for the body. Eventually life's changes took both Sarah and Paul along separate paths. Sarah did not see Paul again for many years.

After several years of building her physical yoga practice, Sarah decided it was time to face her mind. She decided to do a ten-day vipassana retreat in Asia. Despite the very flexible muscles and wide range of motion that her yang practice gave her, Sarah found sitting for an hour several times in a day to be excruciating. She was amazed how poorly prepared she was physically for the practice of meditation. It is hard to face your mind when all you can hear is your body screaming.

Fortunately Sarah's path again crossed Paul's. She returned to the yin practice she had dropped a few years before. By this time, Paul had begun explaining the benefits of the practice. This understanding of the physical and energetic benefits convinced Sarah she needed to stick with both the yin style and the yang style of asana practice. Her next vipassana retreat was a completely different experience: she was able to sit calmly and go deeper into mindfulness without the distractions she suffered earlier.

Now it was Sarah's turn to share what she had learned. She had already earned a reputation as a skilled and articulate teacher, but she was teaching only the yang aspects of yoga. She decided to share what she knew about yin, as well. Sarah began calling postures on the floor, held for long periods of time, "yin" and the vinyasa practice "yang." Following Sarah's lead, when Paul found a publisher for his manual, he renamed it Yin Yoga. As we have seen, this was not the birth of Yin Yoga by any means, just the birth of a name[50].

During the time that Sarah was discovering the yin side of yoga, she and her husband had been investigating Buddhist mindfulness.[51] Sarah began combining this aspect of the practice with the physical and energetic work of yoga. Sarah's teaching is distinct from Paul's; she interweaves the insights and practices of yoga and Buddhism into an integral practice to enliven the body, heart, and mind. Sarah's website[52] describes her teaching:

Her yoga style blends both a Yin sequence of long-held poses to enhance the meridian and organ systems, combined with a flow or Yang practice, influenced by Viniyoga, Ashtanga, and Iyengar teachings. Sarah feels that enlivening the physical and pranic bodies, as well as learning to open to our emotional difficulties is paramount for preparing one to deepen and nourish insights into one's essential nature—a natural state of awareness.

Sarah continues to travel with her husband, Ty, offering Insight Yoga worldwide. Insight Yoga interweaves Yin/Yang Yoga, with Buddhism and spiritual psychology. Sarah is also the co-founder of Metta Journeys, a service-oriented organization that offers yoga retreats internationally to help women and children in developing countries. In 2010, Sarah and Ty created an institute to allow students to delve even more deeply into her Insight Yoga philosophy and practice. The Insight Yoga Institute offers two ten-day retreats in a two-year program in both the US and Asia and is a 500+ hour Yoga Alliance endorsed certificate program.

NOTES

1. This concept of the Dao is not unique to China; it has been observed in many cultures throughout history. In India it is *Dharma*, the law that holds the universe together. In ancient Egypt it was called *Ma'at*: her cosmic balance would weigh a man's soul at the end of his days; without Ma'at, there would be only chaos. *Logos* served a similar role for the Greeks: it is the underlying order of the universe.

2. A *vinyasa* is a sequence of postures or asanas that flow smoothly from one to the next. It literally means "to place in a special way."

3. The term "yogi" is "a person who practices yoga" and so is gender neutral. When we wish to specifically refer to a male practitioner, the term "yogin" is used, and for a female practitioner, "yogini" is used.

4. The yogis have similar words for yin and yang, *tha* and *ha*, which together form the word *hatha* after which the well-known school of yoga is named.

5. Individuation is the process of making the individual whole psychologically. In this respect it is similar to several yogic concepts, but individuation is applied in the psychological realm, whereas yoga was applied to the spiritual realm. We need both: as Georg Feuerstein once said, "Enlightenment is no substitution for integrating one's personality."

6. Robert Johnson is a Jungian analyst, lecturer, and author of several illustrative books on Jungian concepts and relationships, such as *He*, *She*, and *We*. He has studied in Switzerland at the Jung Institute and in India at the Sri Aurobindo Ashram.

7. From *Owning Your Own Shadow*, by Robert Johnson, p. 78.

8. Elastic materials return to their original shapes once the stress upon them ends. Plastic materials retain the new shape.

9. In other words, children do not need to do Yin Yoga for physiological reasons. However, some kids may benefit from some of the energetic or meditative aspects of the practice, but it is not really recommended for children. Childhood is a time to play, not sit still and meditate.

10. Brief can mean five or eight breaths or up to one to two minutes.

11. Tetany is an involuntary cramping of a muscle. Think of the last time you had a cramp: cramps are not fun! We really don't want to deliberately cramp up our muscles by keeping them contracted for long periods of time.

12. This theory applies beyond the tissues of our body. We need to have stress, and then rest, in all areas of our life in order to be healthy, including our relationships, mental abilities, and even our immune systems. For example, cancer patients rarely get colds before getting cancer. Their immune systems were not exercised by colds and thus were weaker than the immune systems of people who did get colds regularly. We need to appropriately stress our immune systems in order for them to be strong. But we also need rest.

13. If you are curious about the above examples, feel free to start a discussion in the www.YinYoga.com Forum discussion board.

14. See Michael Alter, *The Science of Flexibility* (Champaign, IL: Human Kinetics, 2004).

15. Arguably around 200 C.E. and mythically attributed to the sage Patanjali.

16. Yoga Sutra, pp. II-29 and II-46.

17. Georg Feurstein, *The Shambhala Encyclopedia of Yoga* (Boston: Shambhala, 2000), p. 121.

18. The Pradipika actually describes other positions, which are used for pranayama or mudra work, but these are not listed specifically as asanas.

19. Hatha Yoga Pradipika, p. I-43.

20. Ibid, p. I-35.

21. Ibid, p. I-19.

22. Ibid, pp. II-7 and 8.

23. Feurstein, *Shambhala Encyclopedia*, p. 105.

24. Krishnamacharya's famous students included B.K.S. Iyengar, Pattabhi Jois, and his son T.K.V. Desikachar.

25. In the Yin Yoga style Supta Virasana is called Saddle pose.

26. B.K.S. Iyengar, *Light on Yoga* (New York: Schocken Books, 1979), p. 125.

27. Daoism is often spelled "Taoism" but since it is pronounced more with a "d" than a "t" sound we are adopting the former spelling.

28. *Dao* is the way, or path. *De* means "virtue;" however, it is often translated as "power"; *Ching* is a book or story.

29. This philosophy is echoed in many teachings east of Iran, but in the West, it is blasphemy. In the West, Man is part of creation and we are not part of the Creator: we sit apart from the Creator. This is a dualistic view of creation. In the East, for the most part, the philosophies espouse the non-dualistic view that Man is part of the Creator and that the Creator is within each of us.

30. We are using Eva Wong's definitions for the five systems of Daoism. If you would like to further study this fascinating field, you could start with her book *Taoism*.

31. Eva Wong, *Shambhala Guide to Taosim* (Boston: Shambhala, 1996), p. 173.

32. The lower tan-t'ien is found in the belly, around the navel. It is the home of the generative energy. Thanks to the fire (yang energy) found in the stomach area, the generative energy is transmuted into vital energy. The middle tan-t'ien is located in the chest region. Here the vital energy is transmuted into spirit energy. The upper tan-t'ien, located where the Indian yogis place the sixth chakra, is between the eyebrows. Here the spirit energy is gathered, stored, and eventually merged with the original vapors of the Dao itself.

33. This practice is described in detail at the end of chapter two.

34. Called the Marco Polo of the inner world of China.

35. Note the capitalization of the first letter here. To distinguish between the Western use of a word and its close, but not exact, Daoist equivalent, we will capitalize the Daoist terms.

36. Wong, *Shambhala Guide to Taoism*, p. 212.

37. Curiously, there is an understanding in Indian yoga that one is born with just enough breaths to allow us to live to be 108 years old. However, if we breathe too quickly, we will use up our allotment of breaths too soon, and we won't reach that nice ripe age. Slowing the breath down has been recognized by many people as a key to longevity—just as with the turtle. We will return to this topic in chapter two when we look at breath work during Yin Yoga.

38. Paulie Zink loves to say, "To flow with the Dao, move like a cow!"

39. Wong, *Shambhala Guide to Taoism*, p. 223.

40. According to Paulie Zink, the prisoner's name was Kou Sze. When he was released from prison he became a bodyguard. One of his students, Ken Tak Hoi was so good that he served at the imperial palace and later opened up his own bodyguard school, eventually relocating to Hong Kong. Ken Tak Hoi's protégé in Hong Kong, Cho Chi Fung, was the uncle of Cho Chat Ling.

41. This was not the first time that monkeys had inspired a martial arts practice. Several other forms of Monkey kung-fu are described on Wikipedia.

42. Do a search on YouTube for "Paulie Zink" and watch him move. You will also be amazed at Paulie's grace and fluidity.

43. Sometimes this form of yoga was referred to as "Dao Yin." There are many different styles of Dao Yin and it has a long history of its own, just as Hatha Yoga has a long, rich history. Paulie's teaching is just one of many branches of the Dao Yin tree.

44. Learn more about Paulie Zink at www.pauliezink.com.

45. We will look more deeply into Paul's realizations in chapter 6.

46. Tidbits of Dr. Motoyama's life are sprinkled throughout his books. Curious readers can find more details in the book *Awakening of the Chakras and Emancipation*. Here you can learn about the rigor of Motoyama's early training and the awakening of his many *vibhutis*, or powers: his ability to see the energy fields, his ability to influence and correct faulty energy, to heal both those close to him and those in need far away. For a brief biography, visit: http://www.cihs.edu/cihs/Dr_Motoyama_bio.htm

47. Her name was Kinue Motoyama and she was the founder of the Tamamistsu Jinja religious organization. She was also called Myoko no Kamisama.

48. The American institute is called the California Institute of Human Science (CIHS) and is located in Encinitas, California. Paul received an honorary doctorate from the CIHS in 2005.

49. You can learn much more about Paul Grilley at his website, www.paulgrilley.com.

50. The idea of holding a pose for a long period of time, which Paulie rediscovered during the development of his own form of Daoist Yoga, has existed since before the ancient Hatha Yogis first practiced asana. Other physical practices, such as gymnastics and dance, have also used the same form of practice to help open the body. For example, ballerinas often develop openness in their hips by sitting in splits for long periods of time.

51. Their Tibetan teacher, Tsoknyi Rinpoche, influenced them greatly as did their Zen teacher, Toni Packer. Sarah also credits Jennifer Welwood, Lama Tsultrim Allione, Lama Pema Dorje, and Stephen Batchelor with having a great influence upon her.

52. http://www.sarahpowers.com/approach.html

chapter two The Practice of Yin Yoga

How we practice is much more important than what we practice. Too often, yoga students force themselves into contorted positions with no regard for whether what they are doing is helping them or hurting them. Their egos are in control, and the ego wants to look good in front of others. Yoga was never a competitive sport:[1] it is an inward practice designed to build awareness, non-attachment, equanimity, and contentment. We do not use the body to get into a pose, we use the pose to get into the body. Practiced correctly, yoga can provide all the physiological benefits while offering the deep inner calm and insights treasured by the yogis of old. We simply have to practice mindfully, with attention and intention.

In the next few sections, we will look at this question of *how* to practice Yin Yoga. Then we will be ready to look at the asanas most commonly used in Yin Yoga. There are not nearly as many asanas required in the yin style of yoga as are found in the more active practices. There are perhaps three dozen postures at most (excluding variations). We will discover the most common poses and see them in detail, including their variations, options, and some contraindications.

Then we will investigate several flows, which are simply a linking together of asanas in a logical sequence with a central theme or purpose in mind. The asanas presented will not exhaust the possible poses one can do in Yin Yoga, and the flows will be even less exhaustive.[2] While Yin Yoga generally targets the lower body, it is possible to apply the philosophy to any area. We will look briefly at some upper body Yin Yoga practices as well as special conditions that Yin Yoga may assist with, such as pregnancy, knee issues and lower back disorders.

▷▷▷ Before embarking on this practice, please make sure you are able to do so safely. Check with your doctor or health care professional before starting any yoga practice. The guidance given in this book is not meant to replace medical advice. While care has been taken in compiling the guidance in this book, we cannot take responsibility for any adverse effects from your practice. When you are unsure of any aspect of the practice, or feel unwell, seek medical advice. Please read the contraindications for each pose before you try it, and please note the many options available to make each pose more accessible. Practice with both intention and attention.

How to Practice Yin Yoga

> Having seated (himself) in ... a room and free from all anxieties, (the student) should practice yoga, as instructed by his guru.[3]

Straightforward advice. "What type of room?" you may wonder. Well the room is easy to come by; simply find for yourself:

> ... a small room of four cubits square, free from stones, fire, water and disturbances of all kinds, and in a country where justice is properly administered, where good people live and food can be obtained easily and plentifully ... The room should have a small door, be free from holes, hollows, neither too high nor too low, well plastered with cow dung and free from dirt, filth and insects.[4]

Well, finding a place like this can't be too difficult, can it? Cow dung is plentiful and probably available at your local Safeway. Justice is universal today. That is all easy ... but what the heck is a cubit?[5]

The above teaching shows us that advice given in ages past may not be the best for us in our current age. Having a good teacher who can interpret the teachings and intentions of the gurus of ages past and bring the teachings to us in a modern manner is invaluable. In India, where the days were very warm and sometimes scorchingly hot, the asana practices were often done very early in the morning. Is that the best time to do Yin Yoga? Let's examine this question.

When to Practice Yin Yoga

There absolutely are no absolutes. The question of when to practice Yin Yoga has no single answer. We have many options for when to practice Yin Yoga, depending on what we would like to achieve through our practice. It comes down to our intention.

We could do our yin practice:

▷ When our muscles are cool (so they don't steal the stress away from the deeper tissues)

▷ Early in the morning (when the muscles are more likely to be cool)

▷ Later in the evening before bed (to calm the mind before sleep)

▷ Before an active yang practice (again, before the muscles become too warmed up)

▷ In the spring or summer (to balance a natural yang time of year)

▷ When life has become very hectic (to balance the yang energies in our lives)

▷ After a long trip (traveling is very yang, even if we are sitting down a lot)

▷ During a woman's menstrual cycle (to conserve energies).

We could set an intention to maximize the physiological benefits of our Yin Yoga practice—to work into our joints and connective tissues. Or we could intend to maximize the emotional or psychological benefits—to deepen our mindfulness practice. Or we could decide to work on our energy body—to increase the flows of energy or remove blockages. Depending upon which intention we set, the best time to practice will vary.

Physiologically, Yin Yoga targets the deeper connective tissues. If the muscles are warm and active they will tend to absorb most of the stress of the pose, so we want the muscles to be relaxed. When we do Yin Yoga early in the morning, the muscles have not yet woken up; this is why we sometimes feel stiff when we first wake up.[6] In the same way, doing our yin practice before an active yang practice allows the stress to settle deeper into our tissues.

By the end of the day our muscles have been warmed up and are at their longest. The physical benefits of a yin practice will be fewer at this time;

however, the psychological benefits may be greater. The daytime is yang: a yin practice before going to sleep may balance this energy. Similarly the spring and summer are yang times of year. When life is busy or when we spend many hours traveling, these are yang times. Balance is achieved when we cultivate yin energies.

However, a yin practice is not recommended when we have already been very placid. After sitting at a desk for eight hours in the dead of a dull winter's day, a more active practice may create balance much better than a yin practice. Listening to your inner guide may give you the best answer to the question: is this a time for yin or yang?[7]

Before You Practice

Even though Yin Yoga is considered a gentler practice than its yang brother, it is still important to consider the most common precautions. Please note this is not an exhaustive list. If you have questions, please talk to a teacher or your health care professional.

▷ If you are pregnant or have serious health concerns such as joint injury, recent surgery, epilepsy, diabetes, or any cardiovascular diseases (especially high blood pressure), be sure to discuss your intention to practice yoga with your health care provider.

▷ Don't wear perfume or cologne when you practice. Deep breathing is part of the practice and you do not want to be deeply inhaling these fumes.

▷ Do not eat anything for at least one to two hours beforehand, and no big meals at least three hours before you practice. (For yang practice you would extend the waiting times before practicing.)

▷ Before you begin it is nice to have a shower. Empty your bowels and bladder. These are all part of the normal morning ritual, which means you won't be doing your Yin Yoga practice right after rolling out of bed. Give yourself at least thirty minutes after rising before starting any yoga practice.

▷ If you are already physically exhausted, keep the practice very brief and gentle.

▷ Avoid practice if you have had a lot of sun that day. Prolonged sunbathing depletes the body—let it recover before stressing it further.

▷ Remove wristwatches and anything metallic that makes a complete circle around the body.[8] If practical, remove glasses, too.

▷ Wear loose, comfortable clothing so that the body is not restricted.

▷ You will not generate heat internally, so feel free to wear extra layers of clothes and socks. Keep the room a little warmer than normal.

▷ Have cushions, blocks, and blankets handy for padding and to sit up on for most forward bends and meditation.

▷ Remove obvious distractions: unplug the phone, put out the cat, tell family members that you need some quiet time.

▷ Avoid drafts and cold flowing air.

Above all, practice in a relaxed manner. If you have something to do right after your practice, decide to finish earlier than necessary, so you don't feel rushed at the end. Don't expect to have a "great practice;" that kind of expectation can be counter-productive. Expect to do the best you can, and just be present to what arises.

The Three Tattvas of Yin Yoga Practice

A *tattva* is the reality of a thing, or its category or principal nature. Sarah Powers offers us three very simple and effective principles for the yin practice:

1. Come into the pose to an appropriate depth.

2. Resolve to remain still.

3. Hold the pose for time.

Remembering these three principles as you practice will simplify everything. The first principle, which applies to any yoga asana, is often called "playing our edges."

Playing Our Edges

The first principle of Yin Yoga is this: every time you come into a pose, go only to the point where you feel a significant resistance in the body. Don't try to go as deeply as possible right away. Give your body a chance to open up and invite you to go deeper. After thirty seconds or a minute, usually the body releases and greater depth is possible: but not always! Listen to the body and respect its requests.

Consider your will and your body as two dancers, moving in total unison. Too many beginning and even experienced yoga students make their yoga into a wrestling match—the mind contending with the body, forcing it into postures that the body is resisting. Yoga is a dance, not a wrestling match.

The essence of yin is yielding. Yang is about changing the world; yin accepts the world as it is. Neither is better than the other. There are indeed times when it is appropriate and even necessary to change the world; other times it is best to just allow things to unfold. Part of the yin practice is learning this yielding.

This philosophy is reflected well in a prayer, which has uncertain roots. It has been circulating the world for perhaps one hundred years[9] and speaks to this very challenge of balancing yin and yang:

> *God grant me the serenity to accept the things I cannot change*
> *Grant me the courage to change the things I can change*
> *And grant me the wisdom to know the difference.*

Harmony or balance in life comes from this wisdom, which must be earned and learned through our own experience. Our first tattva is the opportunity to gain this wisdom. Listen to your body and go to your edge. When and if the body opens and invites you in deeper, then accept the invitation and go to the next edge. Once at this new edge, again pause and wait for the next opening.

In this manner we play our edges, each time awaiting a new invitation. We ride the edges with a gentle flowing breath, like a surfer riding the waves of the ocean. The surfer doesn't fight against the ocean; she goes with it.

When you come into the pose, drop your expectations of how you should look or be. There is a destructive myth buried deep inside the Western yoga practice—that we should achieve a model shape in each pose. That is, we should look like some model on the cover of a yoga magazine. To dislodge this myth we should adopt this mantra:

> *We don't use our body to get into a pose,*
> *we use the pose to get into our body.*

Once you have reached an edge, pause. Go inside and notice how it feels. The pose is working if you can feel the body being stretched, squeezed, or twisted.[10] Another mantra to adopt in our practice is:

If you are feeling it, you are doing it.

You don't need to go any further if you are already feeling a significant stretch, compression, or twist. Going further is a sign of ego; staying where you are is embracing yin.

This is not an excuse to stay back and not go deep into the posture. When we play our edges we come to the point of significant resistance. This will entail some discomfort. Yin Yoga is not meant to be comfortable; it will take you well outside your comfort zone. Much of the benefit of the practice will come from staying in this zone of discomfort, despite the mind's urgent pleas to leave. This, too, is part of the practice.

As long as we are not experiencing pain, we remain. Pain is always a one-way ticket out of the pose—a signal that we are tearing the body or close to it.[11] Burning sensations, sharp stabbing, or tingling electrical-like pains are definite no-no's and warrant that you come out of the pose immediately. Dull, achy sensations are to be expected, however. No teacher can know what you are feeling, so be your own guru at these times and develop your wisdom.

The Goldilocks' Position

Remember the tale of Goldilocks and the Three Bears? Goldilocks found the momma bear's bed too soft and the papa bear's bed too hard, but the baby bear's bed was just right. The Goldilocks' Position is not a posture, but rather advice about how deep we should go in our poses to ensure we achieve optimal health. Note, we are not talking about optimal performance! That is the trade-off we have to understand: whenever we practice yoga, we need to be clear about our intentions—are we striving for optimal health, or are we working toward some performance goals? Athletes, dancers, and gymnasts may well be trying to maximize their range of motion, but this does not mean that they are getting healthier. Quite the contrary: many athletes and dancers have significant joint issues in later life because they dangerously stressed their bodies to obtain maximum performance when they were younger.

The optimal position for health is the Goldilocks' position: not too much and not too little. This can be shown graphically: on the following page is a classic n-shape curve that illustrates the danger of being outside the optimal bounds. If we apply too little stress to our tissues, they atrophy. All living things require some stress to be healthy! If we apply too much stress, however, tissues degenerate. There have been many scientific

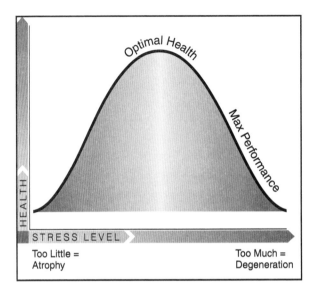

studies verifying the n-shaped curve shown above.[12] To obtain maximum health, we need to find that place where the tension in our poses is "just right"—not too deep, which creates degeneration, and not too little, which promotes atrophy.

Our edges are not only physical—we have emotional and mental edges, too. You may be unconsciously holding back from going deeper to avoid a flood of painful memories, thoughts, or feelings. You may not be ready for these yet. Honor your edges wherever they appear and, above all, notice them!

Playing the edges is not always a "go further" process. Often we go forward, pause, maybe back up a little, wait, and then go again or just stop there. Our edges are always changing, and today may be quite different than yesterday. Our bodies change. Some days we retain more water in our tissues than other days.[13] Water retention affects our flexibility. Our edges will not be in the same place every day. Accept these changes and just take what is offered. Acceptance: that is the essence of yin.

Resolving To Be Still

The second tattva of the Yin Yoga practice is stillness. Once we have found the edge, we settle into the pose. We wait without moving. This is our resolution, our commitment. No matter what urges arise in the mind, no matter what sensations arise in the body, we remain still.

There are two exceptions to this advice. First, we move if we experience pain or if we are struggling to stay in the pose. The second exception is that we move if the body has opened and is inviting us to go deeper. Unless one of these two arises, we remain still.

There are three kinds of stillness we seek:

1. Of the body, like a majestic mountain
2. Of the breath, like a calm mountain lake
3. Of the mind, like the deep blue of the sky

Stillness of the Body

The body becomes as still as a great mountain, unaffected by the winds and dramas swirling around it. Clouds come and clouds go, rains pelt and snows melt, but the mountain remains.

Stillness in the body means the muscles are inactive. Every time we move, we engage our muscles. The muscles naturally want to take any stretch in the body. One of the muscles' jobs is to protect the joints. Only if we keep the muscles very quiet can we allow the effect of a deep stretch to sink into the joints.

When we move, we require energy, which is obtained by breathing. When we move, we affect the breath. Stillness of the body leads to a quieting of the breath.

Stillness of the Breath

Stillness here does not mean cessation. The breath becomes quiet, unlabored, and gentle. Like the surface of a mountain lake, unruffled by wayward breezes, the breath is calm. A calm breath is regular and even, slow and deep, natural and unforced.

Some students prefer a soft *ujjayi* breath during their yin practice[14]. This is perfectly okay, as long as it is soft. The harsher ujjayi found in the yang practices may create waves on the surface of the lake. A soft, rhythmic, ocean sound of the breath will assist with calming the mind.[15]

The breath need not be shallow or short, but it must be regular and unforced. You may try to extend the breath to four seconds or longer on each inhalation and exhalation. There may arise natural pauses between the inhalations and exhalations. In the pauses between the breaths is the deepest stillness. Allowing the breath to be long, even, and deep is part of allowing this stillness to arise.

Once the breath has become quiet, the deepest stillness arises.

Stillness of the Mind

Long ago yogis noticed that controlling the mind by using the mind is really hard. That is the Zen practice of the Samurai warrior and requires tremendous willpower. However, there is a back door to the mind, and that is through the breath. The mind and the breath are like two fish in a school; when one moves, the other moves. If our mind is agitated, our breath is short and choppy. If the breath is short and choppy, the mind becomes agitated. However, if we slow the breath down and breathe more deeply, the mind also slows down.

The sky is always with us. Clouds may block our view, but we know with certainty that, behind the clouds, the deep blue sky is there. The sky is a metaphor for our true nature. We rarely see who or what we are because so many thoughts and distractions prevent us from seeing clearly what is really there. This vision of our true nature is possible only when the clouds of thoughts have drifted away; stillness of the mind is required for this clarity. Stillness cannot be forced; stillness here must arise spontaneously of its own accord. We can, however, create the conditions for this arising.

To still the mind, the breath must be calm. To calm the breath, the body must be still. When these conditions have been met, deep awareness is possible. This state can be achieved only by commitment and dedication. Commit to stillness and allow whatever arises to be just what it is.

Holding for Time

When we have arrived at our edge, once we have become still, all that is left to do is to stay. The yin tissues we are exercising are not elastic tissues. They do not respond well to constant movement: they are plastic tissues, which require long-held, reasonable amounts of traction to be stimulated properly.

Yin tissues don't respond well to maximum stresses held for a short time. Paul Grilley noticed that basketball players, who jump up and down, placing tremendous loads upon the ligaments of their feet, do not develop fallen arches. Their arches don't fall because the extreme strain is very brief. They are more likely to break bones or tear the ligaments in their feet than to develop fallen arches. However, a one-hundred-pound waitress, who is standing on her feet for eight hours a day, is a prime candidate for fallen arches. She is experiencing a gentle pressure for a long period of time. That is the condition for changing our yin tissues.

Yang postures may be held for as little as five breaths or as long as a couple of minutes, depending upon the style of yoga being practiced. Yang tissues require yang exercise. Yin postures are generally held for at least one minute and sometimes as long as twenty. Yin tissues require yin exercise. It is the long, gentle pressure that coaxes them into being strengthened.

It can be dangerous to mix up these forms of exercise. Yang tissues can be damaged by being stressed in a yin manner. No physical trainer would suggest you try to build stronger biceps by holding a heavy barbell in a half-curled position for five minutes. Muscles need repetitive movement to grow stronger. Similarly, being stressed in a yang manner can damage yin tissues. Repetitively dropping back from standing into the Wheel pose can overwork the ligaments in the lower back, eventually wearing them out. We must make sure we exercise yang tissues in a yang way and yin tissues in a yin way.

How Deep?

Every body is different, but in general, every stress of tissue brings down the tolerance level of that tissue. This is what exercise is all about: we stress tissues to make them weaker, at least initially. Once we release the stress, the tissues recover and become stronger. If we apply too much stress, or hold for too long, or do not allow enough rest, then we are in danger.

The graphs on the following page show how these three variables work together. The curve at the top shows the level of tolerance the tissue can take before becoming damaged. The lower curves show the degree of tension or stress being applied through either repetitive stresses or one prolonged steady stress. The horizontal axis represents time.

Notice how the amount of stress (the top line) that our tissues can tolerate decreases with increased stress and time. Eventually, if we continue to stress the tissues to the point where the two curves cross, injury will occur.[16] However, notice the next graph. Here we see the recuperative effect of rest.

If we stress and then rest the tissue, the tissue's tolerance level increases above what it was before. The key then is to not over-stress the tissue either by having too much stress or holding the stress for too long, but rather to allow the tissue enough time to recover and grow stronger.

Find the Goldilocks' position in all poses, whether yin or yang. Don't go where it is too deep or too much (unless your objective is performance and not health.) Don't stay where it is too little, either. From the physiological perspective, in the Yin Yoga practice, time—not intensity—is the magic

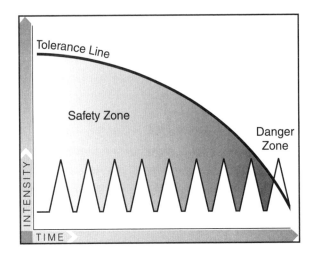

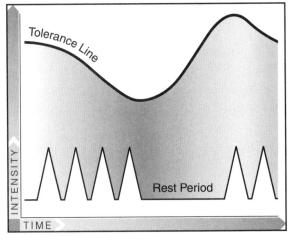

ingredient. To go deeper in Yin Yoga means to hold longer, not necessarily to move further into a pose.[17]

Also remember that you can do too much of anything. Don't hold your Yin Yoga poses so long that you start to exceed your tissues' tolerance levels. Find the middle path!

How Long?

As important as it is to find the right depth, we also have to consider how long to stay in the pose to get optimal health benefits. Again, every body is different, so what might work for a friend could be dangerous for you.[18] Allow yourself time to open up: weeks and even years may be required. In the chapter on asanas you will find some recommended lengths of time to hold each pose: beginners should start at the shorter end of the range, except for those who are already quite flexible and open. The range is just a suggestion. Some students can stay much longer; others may need to come out earlier. It all depends upon your unique circumstances and experience while doing the work.

If you are practicing on your own, use a timer or a stopwatch: three to five minutes may work well for you. If you are just beginning, you may want to start with one- or two-minute holds and work your way toward longer periods. You may find that some postures allow you to remain in the pose longer than others—this is all right: reset the timer and stay longer. Our bodies are not uniformly open. It may be better to stay in a challenging pose, like Saddle, for less time than in an easier pose, like Butterfly. If you are struggling to remain in a pose, come out—regardless of whether the timer has sounded or not.[19]

How Often?

In the yang world we are advised to rest our muscles for at least a day between workouts. The reason for this is to allow the muscles a chance to repair the microscopic damage that occurs during workouts and to allow the metabolic waste products to be removed. To accommodate this rule we choose to work different groups of muscles on succeeding days: the upper body one day, the lower body the next. In the yin world, things are quite different. The waste products produced in our yang workouts are a result of producing energy in our muscle cells. In our yin practice, the muscles are quiet and we do not metabolize our fuels, so there are few or no waste products to get rid of.

During our yin practice we do create microscopic damage to our connective tissues, and we do want time to allow this to heal and become stronger, but studies have shown that we do not have to wait days between practices to allow this healing to take place. One particular study that looked at therapeutic stresses of a damaged joint concluded that "… the clinician's ideal treatment program for a patient with nonosseous, passive joint limitation should be mild stretching, as much as is practical throughout the 24-hour day, 7 days a week, and to start this program as soon as joint motion is allowed."[20]

Remember the arc of aging mentioned earlier? When we are young, we are in the yang time of life and have lots of mobility: what we need when we are young is stability. We need yang exercises. As we age and get older, we move into the yin time of life and we get stiffer: what we need when we are older is mobility. The older we get, the more we should be doing Yin Yoga every day.

Pay attention to how you feel, both during the practice and in the days that follow. If you start to experience pain or tingling, think about what you were doing in your yoga practice (yin or yang!) that may be causing the discomfort and then modify the practice: don't go so deep; don't hold so long. Again, practice with both intention and attention.

The Portable Yin

The yin practice is very portable—you can take it with you anywhere. You don't need a yoga studio or even a yoga mat. All you need is four cubits of space on the floor. That is to say, all you need is enough room to stretch out. You can do these poses while engaging in other activities. While this may not provide you with the deepest benefits (the meditation you get with a dedicated practice will be lacking), you can still affect your tissues physically. Sitting in yin poses while reading or talking on the phone, while eating at the coffee table or watching television, will help open the tightest hips.[21]

One last bit of advice: people love to do things that they love to do. Sounds obvious. Said another way, when you are in balance you will tend to keep doing things that keep you in balance. However, when you are out of balance, you will tend to continue to do things that keep you out of balance! Active people love to do active yoga. Calmer people (a nice way of saying less active people) love to do calming yoga. Don't always practice what you love; practice what you need! Active people probably need Yin Yoga more than anyone else.

Intention and Attention

We are more likely to achieve our goals if we clearly picture what we want to accomplish and keep checking in to see if we are still on track. This comes down to having an intention for our practice, or indeed for our lives, and then paying attention to what we are doing. These two qualities can become another manta for us: what is my intention, and am I paying attention? We will return to this often: let's do everything with intention and attention.

Beginning the Practice

Many students, faced with the challenge of practicing yoga at home, feel overwhelmed by the possibilities of what they could do and are not sure how to proceed. Beginning teachers face the same quandary; what do I do to get started well? Before you even start your practice, it is helpful to think about your intention. Once you have it clear in your mind it's easy to choose the asanas you will do.

Intention

Why are you going to do yoga today? You may never have asked yourself this question, and yet you still feel driven to practice. Why? There are no wrong answers: anything that brings you to your mat is to be respected. But understanding your inner drive will help you focus on your goal, to pay attention.

Reminding yourself of the reason you are doing yoga throughout your practice will help you achieve your purpose. For some, it is to gain health. If this is your reason, remind yourself to feel your state of health as you practice, feel the healing energies flowing through you. You will heal faster when you remember this intention. For others, the purpose is to strengthen the body or open it up.

Perhaps you are going through a very hectic time in your life right now, and you need to slow down. That will be your goal today: balance. Some people do yoga as part of a meditation practice or just because they know they will feel better after they are finished.

These are all perfectly valid reasons for doing yoga. But there can be more—we can set an intention beyond our own benefit. This can be done at the beginning of each and every practice. Certainly all the other physical, psychological, and emotional benefits will still be there, but we can achieve even more. Prayer for centuries has been used in the same manner; we dedicate our efforts to a greater purpose than ourselves.

In the yoga texts, this is called *ishvara-pranidhana*—a surrendering of your efforts to something greater than yourself. As you sit or stand at the beginning of your practice, bring to mind someone or something that needs special assistance, attention, or gratitude. Dedicate your efforts during your practice to that person or thing. This dedication fills you with a resolve to actually do the practice with full *attention* along with the *intention*. When a challenging time comes up in the practice (and it usually will), you will find the extra strength you need because of your dedication.

Invocation

Making an intention into a dedication is sending your energy outward. Sometimes this is not what you need. Sometimes what you really need is to draw energy inward through an invocation. Invoking resources and support from outside the self is a common way to begin a yoga practice.

Invocations can be as simple as chanting "Om" and allowing the vibration to fill our bodies and then linger. Longer chants can also be nice. Chanting is a wonderful form of breath-work. It not only stimulates energy to flow through us but also has a calming, centering effect on the mind. Many students recite chants from the growing availability of kirtan music, such as those by Deva Premal or Wah! and all the various Das brothers.

Not all invocations need to be chanted; you can invoke whatever symbols or energies you relate to. Simply ask in your mind for their support, strength, guidance, or whatever it is you feel you need right now. Your practice is your payment in return.

Opening Meditation

Once you are clear about why you are here today, you are ready to begin. Most beginnings are gentle. A period of meditation is nice. Sit, lie down, or stand in Mountain Pose and meditate. Spend three minutes or more to take inventory and note where you are starting from.

Begin by allowing your awareness to sink into your lower belly. From here notice the rhythm of your own breath. Feel the rising and falling of each inhalation and exhalation. Do not try to change anything. Notice and accept the breath exactly as it is.

After a few breaths, allow your awareness to broaden. Notice other feelings in your body: your weight on the floor, the temperature of the air against your skin, the sounds around you.[22]

After a while, bring your awareness to the heart level and check in with the state of your emotions. This can be difficult, but they need not be big, dramatic feelings. Look closely and don't dismiss anything that appears. The emotion may be as small as boredom. Perhaps there is a little bit of irritation. And contentment can also appear from time to time. The key is just to notice what is arising, without judging yourself for what is there. Don't criticize yourself for being bored or irritated; don't congratulate yourself for being content. Just notice what is happening right now.

After another minute or so, allow your awareness to rise to that point right between the eyes. From here, start to pay attention to the thoughts arising. Don't try to stop them; just watch each new one arise, notice it, and let it float away.

Begin to move your energy. Yin Yoga removes the blockages deep in our connective tissues, allowing the Chi or prana to flow unhindered. In a yang practice we use movement to start this flow of energy, but that engages the muscles, which we try to avoid in the yin practice. In Yin Yoga we can use other techniques.

While you move into, hold, and move out of the postures keep taking inventory. Notice how the practice affects you on the physical, emotional, and psychological levels. Accept whatever you find out and stay curious. There may not be enough time in a short meditation to do all the above practices; don't worry—you will have lots of time during the poses to come back to this.

Flowing

Depending upon what intention you set before beginning the practice, your asanas will vary. Knowing what you want to do makes it a lot easier to decide which postures to choose. For example, let's suppose your intention today is to work your hips. From the list of asanas in the next chapter, you would choose any of the several postures that target or open the hips. If one particular pose doesn't work for you, try another one—that is why several asanas are capable of working a particular area.

In chapter 4 there are several example flows that are designed with specific themes or intentions in mind. There are flows that work the hips, spine, upper body, and legs. There is even one that works the whole body in a yin way. If your intention is to do some energy work, there are two flows you can try; one works the Kidneys and the other works the Liver. If your intention is to have a more mindful, meditative practice, then any of these flows will suffice.

For those just starting out who have little experience with Yin Yoga, there are three introductory flows offered. In time, you will begin to intuitively know which asanas work for you and you will create your own flows.

Beginning Asanas

At the start of our practice we want to ease into the body. Before going deep into a backbend we'll want to do a gentler backbend to prepare. The same applies to forward bends or twists. Open the body with easier postures before going to the deeper openings.

In Yin Yoga we are not actually trying to warm up; we want the muscles to remain cool, so that they are not taking up all the stress of the postures. When the muscles are cool, the stress can go deeper into the connective tissues. There are a few beginning asanas that work well to get us started:

▷ Butterfly: loosens up the hips and spine

▷ Child's Pose: grounding and soothing

▷ Caterpillar and Dangling: loosen up the spine for deeper forward bends

▷ Frog (the Tadpole version): loosens up the hips and upper back

▷ Sphinx: loosens up the spine for deeper backbends and stimulates the Kidney meridian, which helps to support all the other organs.

Each of these postures begins to work a specific area of the body and prepares it for the deeper postures to come. Consider your intentions and which areas of the body you want to work, then choose your first asana to help you work towards your goals. A very flexible student could start her practice with almost any postures if she remembers the first tattva of Yin Yoga: play your edges appropriately. However, there are a few asanas that definitely need preparation before attempting (e.g., even the most flexible students will want to work up to asanas like Snail, the full Seal, and the winged Dragon). Before the Snail, loosen up the neck. Before the deepest backbend like the Seal, do a gentler backbend. Before the deepest hip openers, start with milder versions.

The Butterfly can be a great first pose for almost any practice because it mildly works into the hips and spine: it is a gentle flexion of the spine and hips, a gentle abduction of the thighs and a gentle external rotation of the hips. From here you can go in many directions; deeper hips work, deeper spine work, etc. However, if you practice Yin Yoga in the evening and if you spent your whole day hunched over in front of a computer screen, you may wish to start your practice with a gentle backbend like Sphinx, rather than Butterfly. The point is—choose your first pose deliberately, with consideration of where you want to go, and with where you have just been.

The Ocean Breath

At this point, you are in the flow. You've entered a posture and applied the three tattvas. Now, let's investigate the very yin-like style of breath discussed earlier: the "ocean breath."[23]

There are many forms of breath-work in yoga (called pranayama). Some are very active and stimulating, and there are times when these pranayamas are beneficial. But to turn on the parasympathetic nervous system, which is our rest-and-digest system, we need the slow, deep pranayama known as ujjayi. *Ujjayi* means "victorious breath". A poetic term for this is "ocean breathing."

In Max Strom's *A Life Worth Breathing*, he describes the practice of ocean breathing[24] well: imagine you are trying to fog your sunglasses for cleaning. Try to make this "haahhh" sound on both exhalation and inhalation. At first, do this with your mouth open until you can create the soft sound of the waves coming ashore habitually, without thinking about it. Only then, move to making the same sound with your mouth closed.

Ocean breathing enlivens and expands the lungs, dynamically pulling in fresh air and expelling stale air and stress. It calms the mind and can be very effective for processing grief. If you experience emotions or even some tears from using the ocean breath, simply receive it as a healing experience.[25]

In his book, *The Heart of Yoga*, T.K.V. Desikachar recommends our attention be first focused on the exhalation. Practice watching your out-breath until you know everything about it. Only then, allow your awareness to encompass the inhalations. Then, know everything about the in-breath. Don't worry about the practice of retaining your breath, of holding the breath with lungs full or empty.[26] Instead, allow your ocean breath to lengthen, but don't force it. Surf the breath, and flow with the waves. Desikachar advises that lengthening the breath, while okay, is not the point. The point is to do whatever it takes to stay focused and present, paying attention to the breath. There definitely are physiological and psychological benefits to an extended breath, which we will investigate later.

Here's what it might look like: when you have arrived at that still point in your pose, begin to make the sound of the ocean. Start first with your mouth open. Allow the breath to slow. Count to four as you inhale, pause for one count, count to four as you exhale, and again pause for one count. This totals ten counts, equivalent to six breaths per minute. Next, try it with your mouth closed. Make this into a habit. Whenever you do a pose, start to surf your ocean breath. Eventually, you will be able to do the ocean breath all the time—and not just in your yoga practice.

Next, focus your full attention inward. Notice what it feels like to breathe. Notice everything about your breath and what happens as you breathe. Explore the yin side of your breath.

Linking Asanas

In the yang world, yogis love to create wonderful flows; like a dance we move from one posture into another. There is a rhythm and a logic to these flows: they open the body in stages, prepare us for the more challenging poses, take us to great heights, and allow periods of calm. The yin world is quite different. We hold the poses longer, so we have time for fewer poses in our practice.

We do want to begin the journey with shallower poses before going deeper. Shallow postures naturally precede deeper postures. For example, if you want to work on backbends or stimulate the kidneys, you may wish to start with Sphinx or Saddle Pose. After the mild backbend you will be ready to move into the Seal or Camel.

Many asanas seem to beg to be paired with each other; Shoelace seems to flow naturally, organically into the Swan. Twists easily flow from one side to the other. Straddle folding over one leg easily invites folding over the opposite leg, and then a final fold right down the middle feels very natural, or vice versa.

In the yang styles of yoga, some sort of counterpose to release the tissues follows every deeply held posture. Counterposes move the body in the opposite direction of the previous pose. In the yin style, counterposes are also recommended; however, they do not need to occur right away. It is nice to do some gentle yang movements between postures to relieve any incipient stagnation and to get the energy flowing again. However, it is not necessary to do a counterpose immediately after any particular asana. Feel free to do all your forward bends before moving into backbends. Do all your hip work before moving on to the counterposes. But, don't overdo this—if you are really craving a counterpose at any time, do one!

Counterposes are very logical. Back bends balance forward bends and vice versa. Right balances left. Internal rotation of the hips balances external rotation. Twists can be used to balance almost any pose involving the spine. Sometimes these counterposes are simple movements, sometimes they are long-held poses of their own. Some yang poses seem to be made for when we come out of yin poses: Down Dog feels so good after the Swan. And if you never really cared for Down Dog before, after five minutes of playing with the Dragons, you will quickly learn why the Dog is a yogi's best friend.

By the time you have finished your practice, make sure you have done counterposes for all the deep postures you've held. Some suggested yang counterposes are offered at the end of chapter 3.

Let the body rest for a short time between each pose, especially if it was a very deep one. Respect the body's wishes and take your time between the postures.

Finishing Asanas

In the yang styles of yoga, the teacher will allow a significant amount of time at the end to cool the body down. In the yin practice this is not necessary: we never warmed the body up, but we still want to find a way back to neutrality and balance. Any of the beginning asanas could work well at the end, but a pose often done is the reclining twist. This asana allows the body to fully relax and release. It is one of the most yin-like asanas of all.

The twist in the spine can be directed higher or lower to relieve whatever area was most worked in the practice. Moving the knees higher toward the armpit brings the twist more up the spine by curving the spine forward. Pointing the knees straight away straightens the spine, allowing the twist to be even along its length. Moving the knees downward arches the spine slightly, bringing the emphasis in the twist to the lumbar/sacrum.

Twisting the spine can be done in many orientations. You can do it sitting up or lying down. It is not the only way to end your practice, but twisting does restore equilibrium to the nervous system and gets a lot of the residual kinks out.

Other Considerations

For some students, one side of the body is definitely more open than the other side. Erich Schiffmann has a wonderful suggestion—start your asana on the more open side first. Dr. Motoyama agrees with this advice. Your closed side will watch with amazement at what is happening and will be inspired to open that much as well. Of course, if you don't know which side is more open, it really doesn't matter. But make sure you don't do the same side twice. You may end up with a limp. You laugh! But it happens. One way to make sure that doesn't happen to you is to always start with your right side. That way you will always know that your next side will be the left side.

If you are short of time, do fewer postures instead of holding many poses for less time. It is those last few breaths that give you the most benefit in a pose. It is like that last push-up that strengthens you the most, or that last sugar-filled, creamy doughnut that puts on the most weight. Of course, there are no absolutes, so feel free to do the opposite too; do more poses for shorter holds if you have less time. But shortening the time in the poses moves us away from the real yin nature of the practice. If you have time for only one posture, do the Butterfly.

Finally, be aware of how much time you have allowed for your practice. The opening meditation and poses can take up to fifteen percent of this time, and finishing postures, including Shavasana, may be another fifteen percent or so. That leaves you seventy percent of the time for the key poses you really wanted to get into. Be aware of the time as you flow. Don't shortchange the ending because you got carried away with the fun postures in the middle of the practice. Shavasana is the most important part of the practice, as we will see next.

Ending the Practice

While we do not need to cool down, we do want to restore the body to neutrality. Once we have completed our last pose, it is time for rest and then a transition back to the world we left behind. The rest period is called "Shavasana."

There are two parts to any exercise: stressing the body and resting the body. Most teachers, trainers, and students spend a great deal of time learning how to stress the body in a myriad of ways. Equally important is Shavasana: the relaxation period at the end. Unfortunately, too many students are unaware of the need to balance stress with rest. They may skip their Shavasana, if they are practicing at home or by themselves. Or they may shorten it too much; better to shorten the other asanas and keep the full amount of time available for Shavasana.

Not all forms of rest are equal. One medical study[27] showed that effects of stress were reduced in significantly shorter time by Shavasana than by simply sitting quietly or lying down. It is an active form of relaxing, which sounds like an oxymoron on the surface. Shavasana has been proven to be the most effective form of rest possible. Don't skip it!

When we have finished, we should feel completely balanced. After Shavasana, or even just before it, some quiet pranayama or energy work is often done. Right after Shavasana you may find yourself in a deep, yin-like altered state. Performing some guided breath work can balance your yin and yang energies and wake you up again. Nadi Shodhana, also called alternate nostril breathing, is a good way to balance yin and yang energies.

Closing Meditation

After relaxing and balancing your energy, you may wish to conclude with a brief meditation. This can mirror your opening meditation; you may wish to remind yourself of your intention for the practice and/or conduct an inner inventory. Compare the way you feel now with the way you felt at the beginning. Just note the differences, if any. Do not judge your practice as good or bad.

You may wish to finish with some sort of gesture of completion. Bring your palms together in prayer, leaving a bit of space between the hands to symbolize the space in your heart. Bow down to the floor.

When you rise you may wish to chant something brief. "Om" will suffice, or you can chant *Lokah Samasta Sukhino Bhavantu*.[28] Or, simply end by saying *"namaste"* to all the teachers in your life who have guided you.[29]

For some dedicated yogis, the time after Shavasana is for a full meditation practice. The body is open and strong. Sitting may feel easier, the heart content. The breath is calm right now. It is a perfect time to train the mind.

Transition to Your Next Activity

When the practice is over and everyday life is waiting for you, don't just jump right back into it—savor the quietness for a while. Whatever your next actions are, do them with mindfulness. Allow this heightened awareness to linger throughout the rest of your day. Notice the openness in your body as you move. Smile often and pause frequently. Take time to return to awareness.

Moving Energy

Yoga works on many levels: the physical, psychological, and energetic. How we do our practice can affect our energy body as much as it affects our physical body. There are at least four main ways to stimulate the flow of energy in the body: acupuncture, which relies upon needles inserted in special points along the meridians;[30] acupressure, which stimulates the tissues along the meridian lines (and, associated with this, are all the varieties of massage therapies and asana practices); simple awareness; and directed breathing. In our Yin Yoga practice we do not use acupuncture, but we do apply pressure along our meridian lines to stimulate the flow of energy. When we hold the poses in our Yin Yoga practice we can add two other ways to move energy: awareness and breath.

Simple Awareness

We have mentioned awareness several times already: we practice awareness, we practice presence, when we pay attention to what is actually happening right here, right now in the present moment. When we began our practice with a short meditation, we paid attention to how we were feeling. When we entered a posture and became still, we turned our awareness toward our breath or to sensations that we were experiencing.

Try this little experiment: look at your thumb, and imagine you can feel the energy inside of it. Notice how it begins to warm up, just by focusing there. Continue to focus and feel the thumb for a full minute. The sensation of warmth is not imaginary.

When we bring our attention to a specific part of the body, our parasympathetic nervous system is engaged. When this happens, our heart rate slows down and the blood vessels dilate, allowing more blood and energy to flood the area. We can feel this happening. Simple awareness brings energy to where we concentrate. This is the reason we want to pay attention during our yoga practice to what we are experiencing in the body. We want to enhance the flow of energy through the tissues being exercised, by feeling what is happening there.

A technique used by women during pregnancy to alleviate pain is called effleurage, which means to touch lightly. It is also used sometimes as a precursor to deep massage. Lightly touching the areas of the body that are feeling deep sensations during a Yin Yoga pose will help to bring awareness and energy to that area. You may find that doing effleurage on the area where you feel the pose strongly will diminish the urge to move. Experiment with a light touch, using the tips of your fingers or a deeper pressure using the palm of your hand. For example, in Reclining Twist with the top leg extended out to the side, you may feel a tugging on the outside of the hip. Gently stroke this area with your fingers. Rather than running away mentally from what is happening, bring your awareness right into the sensation. The more you pay attention, the more energy will flow.

Even more powerful than simple awareness is awareness combined with directed breathing.

Directed Breathing

In addition to feeling a particular area of the body, we can also send our breath there. This may sound strange to anyone who has not done this. How can we breathe somewhere beyond our lungs? Take a deep inhalation right now, and notice how your shoulders and abdomen move. This is movement beyond the lungs. When the diaphragm descends, it presses against the stomach and liver. The stomach and liver in turn press onto the lower organs; they also press into the pit of the abdomen. Blood pressure and pulse rate rise on the inhalation and fall on the exhalation. This effect is felt all over the body.

The breath affects every cell in the body, directly or indirectly. Initially, this is something that just happens outside our conscious control. As we practice directing the breath, we can begin to feel the effect of the breath. Later, we can actually increase or enhance this effect deliberately. It is easiest in areas closest to the lungs. Feel the lower abdomen on your next cycle of breath: notice the tension ebb and flow there. Then begin to notice not just the tension but the transfer of energy, too. This combination of both attention and moving the breath to the region doubly increases the energy moving toward the area.

The Hamsa Mantra

On average, twenty-one thousand, six hundred times a day we chant the mantra *Hamsa.* "*Ha*" is the sound of the breath on our exhalations and "*sa*" is the sound of the inhalations. Some traditions reverse this, and the mantra is called "*So'ham*"—we hear "*hmmm*" on the inhalation and a sighing "*sa*" on the exhalation. Iyengar says they are actually combined; every creature creates so'ham on the inhalation (which means "He am I") and hamsa on the exhalation (which means "I am He"). This is called the "*ajapa mantra.*"[31]

While we chant this barely audible mantra with each breath, we can feel energy moving within us. Close your eyes and notice the way your energy state is altered while you inhale and exhale. Experiment with hearing "ham" on the inhalation and "sa" on the exhalation. Does this feel energizing or calming for you? Next, reverse it. Hear "sa" on the inhalation and "ham" on the exhalation. Does this change the energetic feelings?

Like the ocean breath, hamsa breathing can be used outside of your yoga practice. We all have times in life when we are too stoked up and need to relax. The hamsa breath can be useful then. At other times, we need a quick boost of energy, and the opposite breath may be ideal.

Sometimes, even though we can feel the energy flowing through us, it feels unbalanced. After a long yin practice we can feel a bit "out of it." We need to perk ourselves up. Sometimes after a very yang practice, we may feel energized but overly buzzed. We need to calm down. If Shavasana has not brought you back to a calm but alert state, you may need some stronger medicine to come back to balance. Nadi Shodhana may be ideal.

Nadi Shodhana

Nadi means "little river," and it refers to the channels through which prana flows. Nadis are equivalent to the meridians. *Shodhana* means "purification." Thus, *Nadi Shodhana* is a cleansing of the energy passages. Other names for this practice are alternate nostril breathing or *anuloma viloma*.[32] The practice not only cleanses the nadis, it balances the energies on both sides of the body—yin and yang.

The hand position is unique for Nadi Shodhana. The right hand is used, and the middle two fingers are either folded down to the palm or extended so they can rest on the spot between the eyebrows. The right thumb is used to press in on the right side of the nose, closing that nostril. The little finger and ring fingers are kept together and are used to close the left nostril. Since the right arm will be lifted up during the practice, it may get heavy. You can use the left hand to support the right arm.

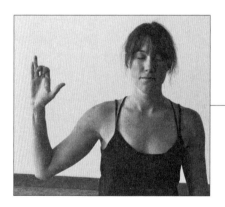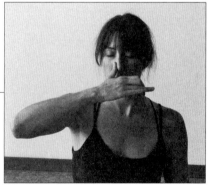

Basic Pattern

Begin with the left side: exhale, and then use the right thumb to press against the right nostril, closing it. Now inhale for a count of four through the left nostril, then release the right side while closing the left side, and exhale for a count of four. Complete the cycle by inhaling on the right side; close it and open the left side, then exhale. Continue with a four-count for eight to twelve cycles. When finished, sit quietly.

Adding Kumbhaka and Lengthening the Exhalation

A more advanced version of Nadi Shodhana keeps the same inhalation timing but extends the exhalation for eight counts. When this is mastered, you may wish to add retentions. Between the inhalation and the exhalation, pinch both sides of the nose closed and retain the breath for four counts. This is antar kumbhaka: retention with lungs full. As you gain experience, you may add bahir kumbhaka at the end of the exhalation, also for four counts. You can try a more advanced, extended Nadi Shodhana practice after a few months with these simple variations, if you experience no difficulties or side effects (visit www.YinYoga.com for a deeper discussion of this).

Orbiting Energy

Ultimately, we would like the energy in our central channel (the *sushumna* nadi or Governor Vessel) to flow freely, unobstructed. Before this happens, we need the meridians flowing beside the central nadi to be open—the ida and pingala nadis. Nadi Shodhana, as just described, is one way to open up both channels. Another way is to mentally circulate energy through these three channels as we breathe and hold our postures. There are several ways to achieve this orbiting of energy.

A Simple Orbit

A simple orbiting of energy begins by feeling the heart center. Sit comfortably and close your eyes. Exhale. Start when the lungs are empty: as you inhale, feel or imagine energy flowing down your spine to the tip of the sacrum. As you exhale, reverse this, and follow the energy as it flows back up to the heart space. Repeat this a few times. Slow the breath down to at least four counts for each inhale and exhale.

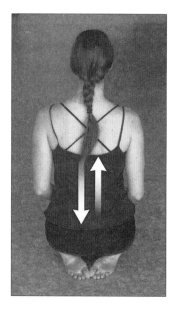

At first, there will be no sensation of anything flowing anywhere. Don't be discouraged; this type of sensing takes practice. For now, just pretend you can feel it. Maybe it would be helpful to imagine someone running a finger along your spine, down from the heart on inhalations and back up to the heart on exhalations.

Once you can follow this flow, even if only in your imagination, add a short pause at the end of the inhalation. The energy now is in the *muladhara* chakra, at the base of the spine. Leave it there for a moment, but bring your awareness to the *ajna* chakra between the eyebrows. Just feel, or pretend to feel, energy there. After a second or so, exhale, following the energy back up to the heart.

Try this for a few cycles. If you can follow the energy without distraction for a few cycles, without losing the flow, add this final variation: continue to pause at the end of the inhalation but add a short pause at the end of the exhalation, as well. By the end of the exhalation, the energy will have returned to the heart space. Leave it there, but bring your awareness back to the muladhara chakra. Feel the perineum[33] and notice the energetic lift there. Hold for just a moment and begin the next inhalation by returning your awareness back to the heart. All of this can be done with the ocean breath. Remember: a four-count inhale, one-count pause, four-count exhale, and a one-count pause.

When we allow energy to descend on the inhalation, we are joining the prana from the in-breath to the apana in the lower belly. When we reverse this, we are joining the apana from the out-breath to the prana in the upper body. This simple work with the breath moves us toward this ultimate goal.[34] We can do this while we hold a pose. All it takes is intention and attention.

Orbiting Energy While in a Pose

Back bends are naturally more energetic than forward bends; forward bends are naturally more calming than backbends. We can practice the simple orbiting of energy in any asana, but when we are in backbends, it feels more natural to pause only at the top of the inhalation, and bring awareness to the ajna chakra. When we are in forward bends, it feels more natural to hold the breath only at the end of the exhalation, and bring our awareness to the muladhara chakra.

When you come into backbends like the Seal, Sphinx, or Saddle poses, orbit the energy as discussed above, but only hold the breath at the end of the inhalation. Bring awareness up to the ajna. Pause for a few seconds and then complete the orbit. Do this for approximately half of the time you are holding the pose. For the second half, simply release and follow the breath's natural rhythm, or come to awareness of the predominant sensation in your body.

When you come into forward bends like the Butterfly, Dragonfly, or Snail poses, again orbit the energy, but this time, hold the breath only at the end of the exhalation. Bring awareness down to the muladhara. Engage your Chi bridge there.[35] Pause for a few seconds, and then complete the orbit.

In any other postures where you are in neither a forward bend nor a backbend, you can continue with holding the breath at the end of both inhalation and exhalation.

A Simple Variation

Now that you have mastered a basic orbit, you may choose to add the side channels. Here we draw the energy down, as before, on the inhalation, but as we hold the breath for a couple of seconds, we send the energy up the left side of the torso, through the heart space, and down the right side, back to the base of the spine. We just hold at the end of the inhalation; there is no retention at the end of the exhalation. On the next cycle, circle the energy up the right side and down the left side while you retain the breath. Cycling the energy through the left and right sides of the body stimulates and balances the flow of energy through the ida and pingala nadis. In all these variations you may wish to add the hamsa, so'ham, or ocean breaths.

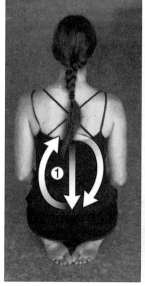
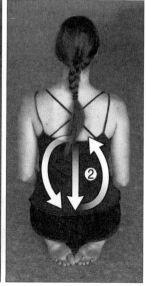

There is a yang variation to the orbiting breath: breathe very *deeply* and hold for a long time with full lungs—this is energizing. In the yin variation, breathe much more quietly, shallowly, and hold only with empty lungs for a few seconds—this is calming.

The Microcosmic Orbit

The term "microcosmic orbit" is a translation of the Daoist term for a full orbiting of energy through the front and back body.[36] In Japanese, it is called "*shoshuten,*" which means a "circling of light."[37] The microcosmic orbit is a way to gather and channel all the stray energies in the body and raise them up from the muladhara to the ajna. This activation of energy is a key preparation for many advanced Daoist practices. Through activating the microcosmic orbit, the reservoirs of the Governor Vessel and Conception meridians are refilled, which means this energy is available to all other meridians and organs. This is perhaps the best way to cultivate health and long life, while at the same time preparing the way to a deep spiritual understanding.

Circulating energy through the microcosmic orbit can be done at any time: prior to asana practice, just before meditation, during the long holds in the yin poses, or even at the beginning of Shavasana as we lay on our backs.

To employ the microcosmic orbit while in Shavasana, bring your awareness to the second chakra on the front of the body. This is the *svadhisthana,* which is about halfway between your navel and pubic bone. Feel, or imagine you

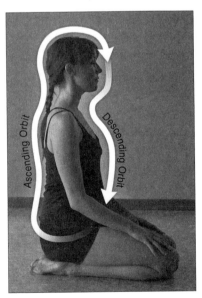

feel, energy there. Exhale completely. As you inhale, follow a flow of energy down the midline of your body, under the pubic bone to the tailbone, and then upward, along the spine, the back of the neck, over the top of your head, and right to the ajna point between the eyebrows. Pause here at the top of the inhalation for two or three seconds. As you exhale, slowly feel the energy descend inside the face and throat. Continue to follow the midline of the body down to the sternum, to the navel, and right back to the svadhisthana. Pause here for two or three seconds before beginning a new orbit.

As you orbit the body, touch each chakra on both the yin and yang sides (front and back) of the body; feel the energy at those points. Two or three minutes of orbiting the energy should be sufficient. When you have finished, release the effort and let the breath be whatever it wants to be. Watch closely how you feel, without reacting to anything.

NOTES

1. Unfortunately, it has recently become just that! There are yoga competitions now, which create an interesting oxymoron.

2. In the YinYoga.com Forum other teachers and students have offered their own favorite flows. Feel free to check these out and add your favorite ones.

3. Hatha Yoga Pradipika, I-14.

4. Ibid, I-12 and 13.

5. A cubit was considered to be the length of a man's forearm, from the elbow to the tip of the fingers, or about eighteen inches. So this would mean you need only about six feet of space (five hundred years ago, apparently, no yogis were over six feet tall).

6. It is generally not a good idea to do any significant exercises immediately upon awakening. The vertebral discs swell up during the night, due to osmosis. If we practice yoga within the first thirty minutes or so after waking up in the morning, we may place too much stress on these ligaments or discs. People with back issues, such as herniated, bulging, or slipped discs, should be especially cautious of flexion first thing in the morning.

7. Listen to your inner voice, but really listen! Most people tend to do what they like, not what they need.

8. Metal circles distort and interfere with electromagnetic energy flow, which is one of the forms of Chi.

9. It has been adopted by Alcoholics Anonymous and is called the Serenity Prayer. Wikipedia claims that the theologian Reinhold Niebuhr originally wrote it in the 1930s or early 1940s.

10. These are the three things we do in a pose: compress, stretch, or twist (shear) tissues. See chapter 6 for more on this topic.

11. We have an unfortunate saying in the West, "No pain, no gain." If you translate this saying into Sanskrit, the language of yoga, it is rendered, "*bullshitihi!*" Instead, in the East we have a better saying, "No pain, no pain!"

12. See Stuart McGill, *Low Back Disorders* (Champaign, IL: Human Kinetics, 2002), p. 32.

13. This is especially true for women, whose bodies change during their monthly cycles.

14. The ujjayi breath is obtained by slightly constricting the back of the throat, the same way as when you try to fog a mirror or glasses with your breath. With lips closed, ujjayi has a "hahhhh" sound on both the inhalation and exhalation. The sound may remind you of the wind in the trees or the waves on the shore. A yang ujjayi may sound more like Darth Vader. Cultivate the softer, ocean-sounding breath.

15. There are several scientific studies showing the benefits of the ocean-breath. These will be covered in chapter 7.

16. The stress that happens when the curves cross can be thought of colloquially as "the straw that breaks the camel's back." It can be a very small stress, such as bending over to pick up your socks off the floor. When we injure ourselves, we like to blame that last movement for causing the injury. In reality it was the accumulation of all the stresses we subjected ourselves to that set up the condition for the injury. Sometimes a student will injure herself in a yoga class and then blame the teacher or the studio. Often Worker's Compensation boards will claim that a worker's job was not responsible for an injury because the worker was at home when she picked up that sock and hurt her back. In both cases it was repetitive strains over time that created the conditions for the injury to happen.

17. More advanced Yin Yoga students do not need to do more and more difficult poses; they simply need to stay in the poses for longer and longer periods of time.

18. Paul Grilley has an instructive mantra that he sings during his classes that reminds us of our uniqueness, "I'm the only one! There is something wrong with me. I must be inadequate in some way. Shanti Shanti Om." This is really how most of us think—that we are the only ones who cannot do this particular pose and therefore we are inadequate and very bad people.

19. Paulie Zink never uses a timer, and as your practice matures you may also find that you will just intuitively know when it is good to stay and marinate and when you should come out. Beginners, however, do not have this inner wisdom just yet, and a timer is quite useful to help us avoid the "coming out too soon" syndrome.

20. This study was conducted by a company that manufactures dynamic splints and can be viewed at http://www.dynasplint.com/pdfs/Contracture.pdf.

21. Thanks to an insidious invention called the chair, our Western backs are very weak and our hips very tight. We constantly lean against the backs of our chairs and couches, which means our back muscles don't have to do any work. To really strengthen our backs, to preserve the natural curve in our lumbar and to open the hips, we should get out of our chairs, slide off our couches, and live on the floor whenever we can.

22. My Yoga Online has several meditations available with these themes: www.myyogaonline.com/videos/meditation/meditation-on-sounds

23. A slow ocean breath while you are holding your poses will reduce stress, activate your rest-and-digest system (the parasympathetic nervous system), improve your heart and lung function, lower your blood pressure, and lead to a healthier and happier life. That seems like a lot to gain from simply breathing, and we will investigate these claims in detail in Chapter Seven.

24. Max Strom, *A Life Worth Breathing: A Yoga Master's Handbook of Strength, Grace, and Healing* (New York: Skyhorse Publishing, 2010), p. 111.

25. Ibid, pp. 112–113.

26. Desikachar warns on p. 60, "…many people think that they can progress quickly along the yoga path by practicing breath-retention techniques, but in fact problems often arise with this emphasis."

27. *Indian Journal of Physiology and Pharmacology: January 2009*

28. This means "May all beings everywhere be happy."

29. *Namaste* is an acknowledgement of the divinity in you and in others.

30. Kids, don't try this at home. It can take years of training to be able to sense where the meridians are and where the specific acupuncture points are along those meridians.

31. *Ajapa* means "unpronounced," thus this is a silent mantra. Another translation is "muttering." See the *Shambhala Encyclopedia of Yoga* by Georg Feuerstein, p. 14, for more details.

32. This means "against the grain."

33. The perineum is the spot at the base of the torso halfway between the anus and the genitals.

34. We are moving a bit beyond the practice of Hatha Yoga now, into the practice of Tantra Yoga, in which the ultimate goal is to awaken Shakti (also known as the Kundalini energy) and send it up along the completely opened sushumna nadi so she can join with Shiva, who is awaiting her at the seventh chakra, just above the crown of the head.

35. Tighten your perineum.

36. In the first chapter, we looked at the translation of *Secret of the Golden Flower*, in which Richard Wilhelm describes the benefits of the microcosmic orbit. It was Wilhelm's work that turned Carl Jung in the direction of alchemy, which the Daoists had been practicing for over a thousand years.

37. This circling of light is an alchemical or transforming process. When the light circles long enough, it crystallizes and the body is transformed. We attain the natural spirit-body, and this body is formed "beyond all heavens." The sages claim in *Secret of the Golden Flower* that the only tool we need to master is this concentration of thought on the circling light.

chapter three Yin Yoga Asanas

The Hatha Yoga Pradipika lists only fifteen asanas and of these, eight are seated positions. Those postures are meant to be held for a long period of time. Today we would call them yin postures. In Paul Grilley's book *Yin Yoga*, he lists eighteen yin poses, along with five yang poses to be used in between them. If you are planning to hold each pose for five minutes, and if you allow a one-minute rest between postures, a five-minute meditation at the beginning, and a five-minute Shavasana at the end, in ninety minutes you will have time for only thirteen poses. There will be even fewer if you are doing two sides or other variations in each posture.

There is not a great need for a lot of postures in the Yin Yoga practice. Paul states in his book, *"The more yin you practice the less variety is needed and the emphasis is placed on a few basic postures."* The next section will list more than two dozen Yin Yoga asanas with the following structure:

▷ A picture of the pose
▷ Benefits of it
▷ Contraindications (reasons for avoiding the pose)
▷ How to get into the pose
▷ Alternatives and options (sometimes with pictures)
▷ How to come out of the pose
▷ Counterposes to be done afterward
▷ Meridians and Organs affected by the posture
▷ Joints affected
▷ Recommended hold times
▷ Names of similar yang asanas
▷ Other notes of interest

The picture of the asana will provide an example of the posture, but please remember that every body is different. The shape is not what's important. To paraphrase David Williams[1]: The real yoga is what you can't see.

The benefits listed in the asana descriptions are not exhaustive but provide a guideline to help you choose when to add a particular asana to your practice. If you wish to arrange your practice time around a particular area of the body or organ that needs stimulation, the advice here may be useful. Combine this knowledge with the information provided on the affected joints, meridians, and organs to structure your flow.

Always check out the contraindications before trying a posture for the first time. Know and respect your limits. If a certain pose is not right for you, there are lots of other ways to work the same tissues. Choose another posture that is more appropriate or accessible from the suggestions offered in the alternatives and options.

The recommended time to hold a pose is subjective. There are guidelines offered, which you should completely ignore if they are not appropriate for you. Some students can remain in the asanas much longer than indicated; others must come out much earlier. Listen to your inner teacher and respect your body's unique needs.

When coming out of a pose there will be a natural sense of fragility—we have been deliberately pulling the body apart and holding it there. The sense of relief is to be expected. Enjoy your practice! Smile when you come out of the pose! Laugh or even cry. Thank the Buddha, Jesus, Allah, Paul Grilley ... shout "Om Namah Shivaya!" Enjoy this moment.

One of the benefits of Yin Yoga is this experience of coming out of the asana. After a deep, long-held hip opener, it may feel like we will never be able to walk again—but be assured the fragility will pass. Sometimes, however, a movement in the opposite direction will help. This is a counterpose, a balancing posture that brings us back to neutral. (Potential yang counterposes are discussed at the end of this chapter.)

Many of these asanas will be familiar to experienced yoga students. However, the name may be different in the yin tradition, and this is deliberate. For example, the yin pose of Swan looks identical to the yang pose of Pigeon, but in the yin practice, we relax the muscles; our intention is to soak deeply into the joints and the deep tissues wrapping them, not the more superficial tissues of the muscles.

There is no consensus in the world of yoga on naming asanas; different names abound. The ones shown here are the names more commonly used, but they are not universal. Where two names are common, both names are given, but we have not attempted to be exhaustive.

The Asanas

This selection will suffice to work all the areas of the body normally targeted in a Yin Yoga practice:

1. Anahatasana (aka Melting Heart)
2. Ankle Stretch
3. Bananasana
4. Butterfly
5. Half Butterfly
6. Camel
7. Cat Pulling Its Tail
8. Caterpillar
9. Child's Pose
10. Dangling
11. Deer
12. Dragons
13. Frog
14. Happy Baby
15. Reclining Twist
16. Saddle
17. Shavasana
18. Shoelace
19. Snail
20. Sphinx and Seal
21. Square
22. Squat
23. Straddle (aka Dragonfly)
24. Swan & Sleeping Swan
25. Toe Squat
26. Yin Postures for the Upper Body

Anahatasana (Melting Heart)

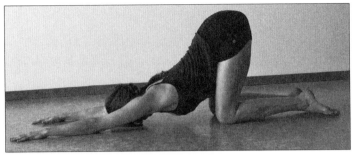

Benefits:
- ▷ A nice backbend for the upper and middle back
- ▷ Opens the shoulders
- ▷ Softens the heart

Contraindications:
- ▷ If you have a bad neck, this could strain it.
- ▷ Be aware of any tingling in the hands or fingers! This is often a sign that a nerve is being compressed, and if we continue to compress it we may permanently damage it. If you feel tingling, adjust the arm and hand positions, or skip the pose entirely.

Getting Into the Pose:
- ▷ On your hands and knees, walk your hands forward, allowing your chest to drop toward the floor. Keep your hips right above your knees. If possible, keep your hands shoulder-width apart.

Alternatives & Options:
- ▷ If shoulder pain prevents the arms from going overhead, move them further apart.
- ▷ If you're flexible, you can bring the chin to the floor and look ahead, but this could strain the neck.
- ▷ If your knees are uncomfortable here, place a blanket underneath them.
- ▷ Toes can be tucked under.
- ▷ The chest can rest on a bolster (allowing the body to relax).
- ▷ You can do this pose with just one arm forward at a time, resting the head upon the other forearm.

Coming Out of the Pose:

▷ Either move back into Child's Pose or slide forward onto your belly.

Counterposes:

▷ Lying on your stomach or in Child's Pose can be nice here. Since this posture is a backbend, Child's Pose is a better choice for a counterpose because it is a mild forward fold.

Meridians & Organs Affected:

▷ Compression along the spine stimulates the Urinary Bladder lines.

▷ If you feel the stretch in the chest, then your Stomach and Spleen lines are stimulated.

▷ This posture can juice up the arm meridians, especially the Heart and Lung lines.

Joints Affected:

▷ Nice compression for the upper back

▷ Mildly stresses the lower spine

▷ Shoulder/Humerus joint

Recommended Hold Time:

▷ Three to five minutes

▷ If resting your chin on floor, the hold may need to be shorter. Carefully watch the sensations in the neck.

Similar Yang Asanas:

▷ Half Down Dog (aka Puppy Dog)

Other Notes:

▷ This pose is nice after a series of lower backbends.

▷ Can be used as a gentle warm up before deeper backbends.

▷ If you feel pinching in the back of the shoulders, you may be reaching a compression point. Abducting the arms (moving them farther apart) may release this.

Ankle Stretch

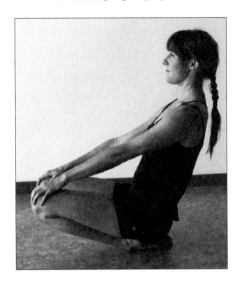

Benefits:

> ▷ Opens and strengthens the ankles

> ▷ Strong stimulation of four meridians flowing through the feet and ankles

> ▷ Great counterpose for squatting or toe exercises

Contraindications:

> ▷ If there is any sharp pain in the ankles, back off. Try placing a blanket or towel under the feet to cushion them.

> ▷ Knee issues may prevent you from sitting on the heels. Placing a rolled-up towel behind the knees may be very therapeutic, but a cushion between the thighs and calves may be required.

Getting Into the Pose:

> ▷ Begin by sitting on the heels. If your ankles or knees complain, this may not be the pose for you.

Alternatives & Options:

> ▷ Leaning back on the hands is the first position (and the least stressful), but beware of collapsing backward. Keep the heart forward, and imagine you are trying to do a backbend.

▷ After a few moments, bring the hands to the floor beside your legs.

▷ Try not to lean away from the knees. Keep the heart open, arching the back forward.

▷ Finally, try holding the knees and gently pulling them toward the chest.

Coming Out of the Pose:

▷ Lean forward and bring your hands to the floor beside the knees. Slowly step one foot at a time back to a push-up position.

Counterposes:

▷ Push-up/Plank/Chaturanga or Crocodile, or any posture that straightens the legs and tucks the toes under

▷ Dangling or Squatting

Meridians & Organs Affected:

▷ Stomach, Spleen, Liver, and Gall Bladder lines are strongly stimulated.

Joints Affected:

▷ Ankle

Recommended Hold Time:

▷ About one minute. Relatively intense, this shouldn't be held for a long time if there is a lot of discomfort. In time you may be able to sit like this for a very long time.

Other Notes:

▷ This is a nice counterpose for many postures that stress the feet, such as Toe Squat, regular Squat, and sitting meditations.

Bananasana

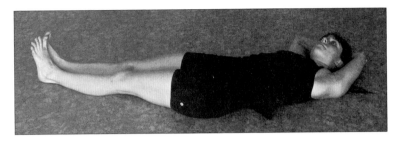

Benefits:

  ▷ A delicious way to stretch the whole side of the body

  ▷ Works the spine in a lateral flexion (side bend) from the iliotibial (IT) band to the top of the side rib cage

  ▷ Stretches the oblique stomach muscles and the side intercostal muscles between the ribs

  ▷ Can even stretch the arm pit

Contraindications:

  ▷ If prone to tingling in the hands when extending your arms overhead, you may need to place a bolster under the arm or simply bring the hands down.

  ▷ If you have lower back issues, you may wish to not go too deep in this pose.

Getting Into the Pose:

  ▷ Lying on your side with your legs together and straight on the floor, reach the arms overhead and clasp your hands or elbows. With your buttocks firmly glued to the earth, move your feet and upper body to the right. Arch like a nice, ripe banana. Be careful not to twist or roll your hips off the floor. Find your first edge. When your body opens more, move both feet further to the right and pull your upper body further to the right, as well. Keep playing this edge. Don't forget to do both sides!

Alternatives & Options:

▷ When your feet are as far to the side as you can get them, try crossing the ankles. Most students feel the greatest stretch by crossing the outside ankle over the inner ankle, but some feel more benefit crossing the other way.

▷ If you feel any tingling in the hands, try supporting the arms with a bolster or resting them across the chest.

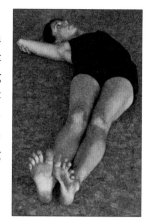

Coming Out of the Pose:

▷ Simply move your legs back to a straight position and bring your arms down.

Counterposes:

▷ Hug the knees to the chest to release the back in a gentle forward fold.

▷ Circle the knees to massage the sacrum and lumbar.

▷ Spontaneously erupt into any pose that feels organic.

Meridians & Organs Affected:

▷ This is a great opening and stretching of the Gall Bladder meridian.

▷ If you raise your arms overhead, you will stimulate the Heart and Lung meridians.

Joints Affected:

▷ Moves the spine and the rib cage in a lateral flexion

Recommended Hold Time:

▷ Can be held for three to five minutes

Similar Yang Asanas:

▷ A lying down version of Half Moon or Blown Palm

Other Notes:

▷ This pose works the iliotibial (IT) band. If you feel tugging at the outside of the hip (the greater trochanter), then you may be working your tensor fascia latae (this is not a drink from Starbucks, but the muscle that connects the IT band to the iliac crest) or gluteus maximus, both of which attach to the IT band.

Butterfly

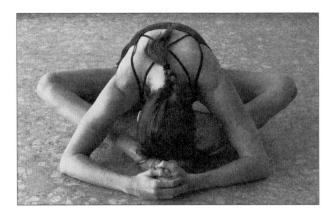

Benefits:

▷ A nice way to stretch the lower back without requiring loose hamstrings

▷ If the legs are straighter and the feet further away from the groin, the hamstrings will get more of a stretch. If the feet are in closer to the groin, the adductor muscles get stretched more.

▷ Good for the kidneys and prostate gland; highly recommended for people suffering from urinary problems[2]

▷ Removes heaviness in the testicles and regulates periods, helps ovaries function properly, and makes childbirth easier [3]

Contraindications:

▷ Can aggravate sciatica. If you have sciatica, elevate the hips by sitting on a cushion, until the knees are below the hips, or avoid this pose entirely. Beware of hips rotating backward while seated; we want them to rotate forward.

▷ If you have any lower back disorders which do not allow flexion of the spine, then do not allow the spine to round: keep the back as straight as you can or do the reclining version.

▷ Avoid dropping the head down if the neck has suffered whiplash or has reverse curvature.

Getting Into the Pose:

▷ From a seated position, bring the soles of your feet together and then slide them away from you. Allowing your back to round, fold forward, lightly resting your hands on your feet or on the floor in front of you. Your head should hang down toward your heels.

Alternatives & Options:

▷ Elevate the hips with a bolster or cushion.

▷ If your neck is too stressed, support your head in your hands, resting your elbows on your thighs or a block.

▷ You can rest your chest on a bolster positioned across the thighs.

▷ Various hand/arm positions are possible: hold your feet, place your hands on the floor in front of you, or relax your arms behind the body.

▷ If the back doesn't like this pose, do the reclining variation; lie down, keeping legs in butterfly.

Coming Out of the Pose:

▷ Use your hands to push the floor away and slowly roll up.

▷ Before straightening your legs, lean back on your hands to release the hips. Then slowly straighten each leg.

Counterposes:

▷ Sitting up or a gentle sitting backbend

▷ Lying on the stomach, which is also a gentle backbend

▷ A spinal lift flow on the back or flow into Tabletop (aka Hammock)

▷ Seated twist

Meridians & Organs Affected:

▷ The Gall Bladder lines on the outside of the legs and the Urinary Bladder lines (these are the same as the ida and pingala nadis) running along the spine in the lower back

▷ If the feet are in close to the groin and a stretch is felt in the inner thighs, the Kidney and Liver lines will be stimulated.

Joints Affected:

▷ Hips and lower spine

Recommended Hold Time:

▷ Three to five minutes or much longer if desired

Similar Yang Asanas:

▷ Baddha Konasana, but without the emphasis on a straight spine or the feet in tight to the groin. In Butterfly, we want the back to round, allowing the head to drop to the heels.

Other Notes:

▷ Can be done after meals, as long as the head does not touch the floor (which would create too much pressure in the abdomen).

▷ If the feet are closer in, tightness in the adductors or lower back may prevent you from folding forward. Move the feet farther away.

▷ If you are tempted to go into a tight butterfly because of your yang training, move the feet away, forming a diamond shape with the legs.

▷ This pose is nice for pregnant women because the legs are abducted, providing space for the belly.

Half Butterfly

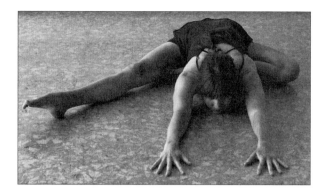

Benefits:

▷ Stretches the lower back without requiring loose hamstrings

▷ Targets the ligaments along the back of the spine

▷ Stimulates the liver and kidneys and aids digestion (when folding over the straight leg)[4]

Contraindications:

▷ Can aggravate sciatica. If you have sciatica, elevate the hips by sitting on a cushion, until the knees are below the hips, or avoid this pose entirely. Beware of hips rotating backward while seated; we want them to rotate forward.

▷ If you have any lower back disorders which do not allow flexion of the spine, then do not allow the spine to round: keep the back as straight as you can.

▷ Beware of any sharp pain in the knees. If you have issues in this area, tighten the top of the thigh (engage the quadriceps), which will close the joint, or bring the legs closer together.

▷ If the bent knee complains, place support under that thigh or move that foot away from the groin.

▷ If the hamstrings protest, bend the straight knee and support the thigh with a blanket or block.

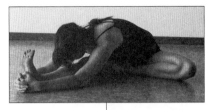

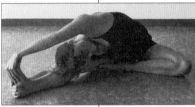

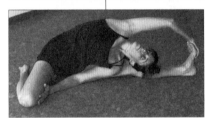

Getting Into the Pose:

▷ From a seated position, draw one foot in toward you and stretch the other leg straight out to the side. Allowing your back to round, fold forward, down the middle between both legs.

Alternatives & Options:

▷ Folding over the straight leg may stretch the hamstrings more.

▷ Reach the opposite hand to the extended foot and/or lower that shoulder to emphasize the side of the spine.

▷ Add a twist to the spine by resting the elbow on the thigh and the head in that hand (or for more flexible students, placing the arm alongside the straight leg) and the other arm behind the back or over the head. Rotate the chest toward the sky. This deepens the emphasis along the side of the ribs and spine.

▷ Place the foot of the bent knee in Virasana (folded backward behind the buttock), but only if knee doesn't complain.

Coming Out of the Pose:

▷ Slowly roll up, pushing the floor away with your hands. Before straightening the opposite leg, lean back on your hands to release the hips. Then slowly straighten the leg.

Counterposes:

▷ Sitting up or a gentle sitting backbend

▷ Flow into Tabletop (aka Hammock)

▷ Windshield Wipers

Meridians & Organs Affected:

▷ Urinary Bladder

▷ If there is a lot of sensation in the groin and inner legs, the Liver and Kidneys will be stimulated.

Joints Affected:

▷ Spine, especially the back and sides

▷ Inner knees, although not as deep of a stretch as Straddle

Recommended Hold Time:

▷ Can be held up to five minutes, with variations added after two or three minutes

Similar Yang Asanas:

▷ Janusirsasana, but we aren't trying to bring the head to the foot; rather, we are bringing the head to the knee. Allow the back to round.

Other Notes:

▷ This can be great for pregnant women because the legs are abducted, providing space for the belly.

▷ Paul Grilley calls the variation with the foot in Virasana the Half Frog.

Camel

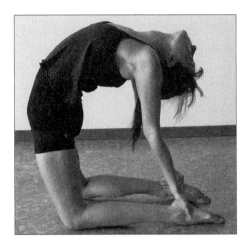

Benefits:

▷ Deeply arches the sacral/lumbar spine and opens the top of the thighs; provides some opening in the ankles

▷ Stretches the hip flexors and opens the shoulders; excellent for drooping shoulders or hunched backs[5]

Contraindications:

▷ Elderly and those with spinal injuries can do this pose.[6] However, seek medical advice if you fit either category.

▷ Without support, the back can spasm, so those with weak backs may want to do only the gentle versions.

▷ If you have any neck issues, do not drop head back; keep the chin to the chest.

Getting Into the Pose:

▷ The easiest way to come into Camel is to sit on your heels, place your hands behind you on the floor, and lift your hips forward. As the hips move forward, your back will arch.

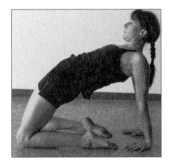

Alternatives & Options:

▷ You may also come into this pose by standing on your knees and holding your hands on your hips. Keeping the hips forward, arch your back. (This may be unsuitable for people with back problems, because there is little support from the hands in this version. Instead, do the hands-on-the-floor version.)

▷ Walking the hands on the floor toward the feet may be unsuitable for people with knee problems because there is more pressure in the knees in the early stages of this variation.

▷ If you're very flexible you may wish to bring your hands to the floor between the feet or move the hands toward the knees. If you're less flexible, the toes can be tucked under and the hands rested on the heels or on a block between the feet.

▷ If the neck is okay, you may lengthen the neck and allow the head to drop back.

Coming Out of the Pose:

▷ There are two ways to come out of this pose: The easy way is to walk your hands backward until you are sitting on your heels again. If your head was dropped back, keep it back while you bring your chest forward and fold into Child's Pose. The second way is to come back up to standing on your knees. If your head was back, lift the chest forward, allowing the head to remain dropped back until the shoulders are over the hips. Then bring the head forward and sit back into Child's Pose.

Counterposes:

▷ Child's Pose is a gentle forward fold, allowing the spine to release.

Meridians & Organs Affected:

▷ The deep compression in the sacrum and lumbar spine stimulates the Urinary Bladder and Kidney meridians, while any feeling of stretch in the top of the thighs and stomach stimulates the Spleen and Stomach meridians.

▷ Sometimes the upper arms and shoulders are stressed, which stimulates the Heart and Lung meridians.

▷ If the neck is dropped back, the thyroid will be stimulated.

Joints Affected:

▷ Spine, shoulders, and ankles

Recommended Hold Time:

▷ One to two minutes at most. This is a very yang-like pose and requires a lot of leg strength in the full posture, or if your hands are on your hips or lower back. In the supported pose, with the hands on the floor or on your legs or feet, you may stay longer, as you can rest on your arms.

Similar Yang Asanas:

▷ Ustrasana (*ustra* means camel)

Cat Pulling Its Tail

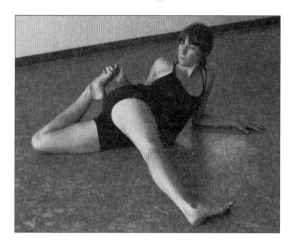

Benefits:

> ▷ A nice counterpose to strong forward bends (such as the Snail or Caterpillar)
>
> ▷ Mildly compresses the lower back
>
> ▷ Opens the quadriceps and upper thighs

Contraindications:

> ▷ If you have lower back issues, go gently. You may not be able to pull the foot away at all.

Getting Into the Pose:

> ▷ Start by sitting with both legs out in front of you. Twist to the right and recline onto your right elbow. Keeping your bottom (right) leg straight, bring your top (left) leg forward and to the side. Bend the bottom leg, bringing that heel toward your buttock. Reach back with your top (left) hand and grab the bottom foot. Pull the foot away from you.
>
> ▷ You may begin lying down. From here, roll onto your right side. Keeping your bottom (right) leg straight, bring your top (left) leg to the side. Bend the bottom leg, bringing that heel toward your buttock. Reach back with your top (left) hand and grab the bottom foot. Pull the foot away from you.

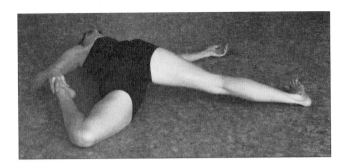

Alternatives & Options:

▷ It's easiest to be propped up on one arm (as shown in the first picture).

▷ It's more challenging to recline and look over the shoulder to the bottom foot. This becomes a reclining twist with a backbend. Try pulling the foot away from the buttock (most will not be able to do this).

Coming Out of the Pose:

▷ Release the bottom foot and roll onto your stomach. Straighten the bottom leg and roll onto your back.

Counterposes:

▷ Hug the knees to the chest to release the lower back in a gentle forward fold. Do this either while lying on your back or in Child's Pose.

Meridians & Organs Affected:

▷ Stimulates the Stomach and Spleen meridians (if the top of the thigh is activated) and the Urinary Bladder and Kidney lines (when the back is arched and twisted).

▷ If you feel a twist through the side of the rib cage, the Gall Bladder meridian is being stimulated.

Joints Affected:

▷ Mostly opens the lumbar and sacrum

▷ The feeling of a twist may indicate that the rib cage is getting some juice, too

Recommended Hold Times:

▷ One minute if done as a counterpose to a forward bend

▷ Can hold for three to five minutes as a reclining twist

Similar Yang Asanas:

▷ Jatharaparivartanasana with a backbend

Other Notes:

▷ If you are actively pulling the foot away, the pose becomes yang-like in nature. In this case, you may shorten the time or release the pressure after one minute.

Caterpillar

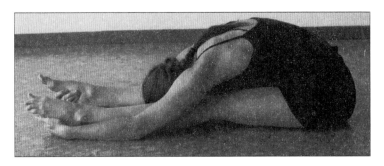

Benefits:

▷ Stresses ligaments along the back of the spine

▷ Compresses the stomach organs, which helps strengthen the organs of digestion

▷ Stimulates the kidneys

▷ Massages the heart

▷ Helps to cure impotency and leads to sex control[7]

Contraindications:

▷ Can aggravate sciatica. If you have sciatica, elevate the hips by sitting on a cushion, until the knees are below the hips, or avoid this pose entirely. Beware of hips rotating backward while seated; we want them to rotate forward.

▷ If you have any lower back disorders which do not allow flexion of the spine, then do not allow the spine to round: keep the back as straight as you can.

▷ If the hamstrings are very tight, the knees should be bent and supported by a bolster, allowing the spine to round.

Getting Into the Pose:

▷ Sit on a cushion with both legs straight out in front of you. Fold forward over the legs, allowing your back to round.

Alternatives & Options:

▷ If your hamstrings are really tight, you won't be able to fold forward enough to allow gravity to draw you down. Bend your knees and place a bolster underneath; allow the back to round fully. If that doesn't work, sit up on more cushions.

▷ If neck feels strained by the weight of the head, support your head in your hands, resting your elbows on the legs or a bolster.

▷ You can rest your chest on a bolster to help relax into the pose.

▷ You can do this pose with the legs up a wall (very nice for people who stand all day).

▷ If knees feel strained, activate the quadriceps (but not all the time!) or keep a small bend in the knees, perhaps with a blanket underneath.

▷ Experiment with hand positions. Rest your elbows on your thighs or the floor, or loosely hold the toes with your hands. No need to pull: gravity will do the work.

▷ If you're very flexible, it might be more challenging if you part your legs just enough that your chest fits between the legs.

Coming Out of the Pose:

▷ Use your hands to push the floor away and slowly roll up.

▷ Once you are up, lean back on your hands to release the hips and then shake out the legs.

Counterposes:

▷ Sitting up or a gentle sitting backbend

▷ Lying on the stomach is a gentle backbend, as is doing a spinal lift flow on the back, or flow into Tabletop (aka Hammock)

▷ A seated twist

Meridians & Organs Affected:

▷ The Urinary Bladder

Joints Affected:

▷ The spine

Recommended Hold Times:

▷ Three to five minutes or more

Similar Yang Asanas:

▷ Paschimottanasana, but here we are not trying to lengthen the spine or stretch the back muscles. Don't try to bring the head to the feet but, rather, round the spine so the head comes to the knees.

Other Notes:

▷ Paul Grilley says this pose is excellent for balancing Chi flow and preparing the body for meditation.

▷ Keep muscles relaxed, especially in the legs.

▷ Make sure the tops of the hips are tilted forward. If the hips are rotating backward, sit on higher cushions and bend the knees more. Fold forward enough that gravity is doing the work, not your muscles. If you are not folding forward, you won't be able to relax completely. Let gravity have you! Surrendering is yin.

Child's Pose

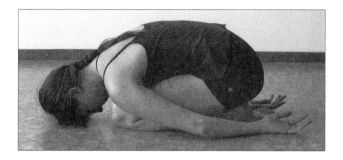

Benefits:

▷ A healing, restful pose—useful any time a break is needed

▷ Gently stretches the spine and is always a nice counterpose for backbends

▷ Gentle compression of the stomach and chest benefits the organs of digestion

▷ Psychologically soothing when feeling cold, anxious, or vulnerable

▷ Can relieve back and neck pain when the head is supported

▷ If the knees are fairly close together, rocking gently side to side can help stimulate the flow of blood and lymph fluids in the upper chest and breast tissues

Contraindications:

▷ If you have diarrhea or are pregnant.

▷ Can be uncomfortable just after eating.

▷ If knee issues exist, you may need to place a towel or blanket between thighs and calves or avoid the pose altogether.

▷ You may need a blanket or other padding under the ankles to reduce discomfort on the top of the feet.

Getting Into the Pose:

▷ Begin by sitting on your heels and then slowly fold forward, bringing your chest to your thighs and your forehead to the earth.

Alternatives & Options:

▷ Can be done with arms stretched forward, which may avoid placing too much pressure on the neck (this reduces the shoulder relaxation).

> If you cannot get your buttocks to your heels, the head will have a lot of weight on it. Support the neck by placing the forehead on hands or on a bolster.

> Allow the knees to be as close together as is comfortable, but they do not have to touch. If there is any uncomfortable pinching in the lower belly and tops of the front hips, separate the knees wider.

> You can do this as a preparation for the Frog by spreading the knees farther apart halfway through the pose, while continuing to sit on the heels.

> Many students love to place a bolster under their chest.

Coming Out of the Pose:

> Use your hands to push the floor away and slowly roll up.

Counterposes:

> A counterpose is not normally needed after this pose.

Meridians & Organs Affected:

> The Spleen and Stomach meridians are compressed while the Kidneys and Urinary Bladder meridians are stretched.

Joints Affected:

> The spine and ankles

Recommended Hold Times:

> As long as you want

> If used as a counterpose, hold for up to one minute.

> If used as a yin pose on its own, hold for three to five minutes. If you cannot get your head to the floor, five minutes may be too long.

Similar Yang Asanas:

> Balasana or Garbhasana

Other Notes:

> This pose can be used as a preparation for Straddle pose or deeper forward bends like Snail.

Dangling

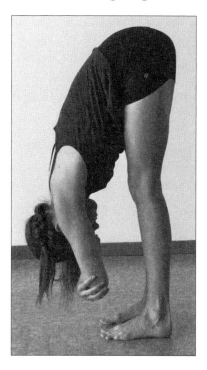

Benefits:

 ▷ Gentle stretch for the lower spine

 ▷ Loosens the hamstrings and warms up the quadriceps

 ▷ Compresses the stomach and internal organs

 ▷ Builds strength in the diaphragm while providing a massage for the abdominal organs

 ▷ Cures menstrual cramps

 ▷ Slows heart rate and rejuvenates spinal nerves

Contraindications:

 ▷ Avoid if you have high blood pressure. (Poses where the head is below the heart can increase blood pressure.) Related conditions that are a problem when blood pressure is increased include diabetes and glaucoma. If you have these conditions you may wish to avoid this pose.

 ▷ If you have low blood pressure, to come out of the pose, roll up to standing slowly or go into squat to avoid dizziness.

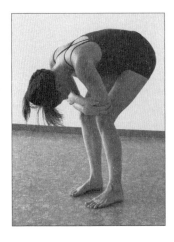

▷ If you have a bad back, bend your knees a lot! You can also rest your elbows on the thighs.

▷ If you have any lower back disorders which do not allow flexion of the spine, then do not allow the spine to round: keep the back as straight as you can and bend the knees a lot.

Getting Into the Pose:

▷ Stand up, with the feet hip-width apart. Bend your knees and fold forward. Clasp the elbows with the opposite hands.

Alternatives & Options:

▷ Bend knees more, which will strengthen the quadriceps and release the back.

▷ Rest elbows against a table, chair, or on the thighs if the back feels strained.

▷ Caterpillar is an easy alternative; sit down with legs straight.

▷ If you do this pose more than once, try it with legs bent the first time and straight the second time.

▷ If you're really flexible, try holding the wrists behind the legs but still with some rounding to the back.

Coming Out of the Pose:

▷ Bend your knees a bit more and release your hands to the floor. Slowly roll up. This is often called Rag Doll.

▷ You can place your hands onto your shins and come up halfway, then fold back down. Do this a couple of times, and when you feel ready, come all the way up with a straight back.

Counterposes:

▷ Squat or any gentle backbend. For example, Upward Facing Cat, lying on stomach, or, while sitting crosslegged with hands on the floor behind you, lift your chest and hips forward.

Meridians & Organs Affected:

▷ Due to the intense stretch along the back of the legs and spine, the Urinary Bladder meridian is highly stimulated.

▷ Great for the liver, spleen, and kidneys[8]

Joints Affected:

▷ The spine

Recommended Hold Times:

▷ Three minutes can be intense. Sometimes this pose is done in two or more sessions of two minutes each, separated by two minutes of Squat.

Similar Yang Asanas:

▷ The yang version is known as Uttanasana, but in the Yin Yoga version the emphasis is not to stretch the hamstrings a lot, but rather to release the lower back. If the legs are straight, it is a nice stretch for the hamstrings, but there is some muscular effort needed. If the knees are bent, it is a great strengthener for the thigh muscles and allows the back to release more fully.

Other Notes:

▷ Ensure the arches of the feet are lifting.

▷ Balance the weight between toes and heels. You can gently sway or wobble, but no bouncing.

▷ Straight legs will stretch the hamstrings; bent knees will strengthen the thigh muscles.

▷ It is more yin-like to bend the knees, bringing the chest to the thighs (you'll receive a stomach massage, too).

▷ Can intermix this and Squat. Eventually, hold both for four minutes or more in total.

Deer

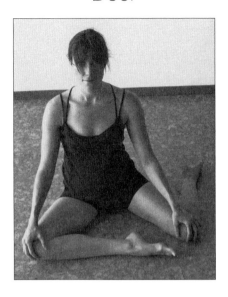

Benefits:
- ▷ A nice counterpose to hip openers or any external rotation of the hips
- ▷ A balanced way to rotate hips, both externally (front leg) and internally (back leg)
- ▷ Improves digestion and relieves gas
- ▷ Helps to relieve the symptoms of menopause
- ▷ Reduces swelling of the legs during pregnancy (until the end of the second trimester)
- ▷ Therapeutic for high blood pressure and asthma

Contraindications:
- ▷ If any knee issues exist, be careful of externally rotating the hip (front knee); keep that foot in closer to the groin. You could support the front knee with a bolster or folded blanket.

Getting Into the Pose:
- ▷ Start by sitting in Butterfly on the floor, then swing your right leg back behind you, bringing the foot behind your hip. Position the front leg by moving the foot away from you. Try to make a right angle with the front knee. Move the back foot away from your hip until you start to

feel like you are tipping away from that foot. Keep both sitting bones firmly rooted to the ground.

Alternatives & Options:

▷ The tendency here is to tilt away from the internally rotating hip of the back leg; make sure both sitting bones are firmly on the floor; you may need to move the feet more inwards, toward the core of the body.

▷ If you're very flexible, you can begin to move your feet away from the hips.

▷ To get a nice stretch to the side body and the back thigh, twist around toward the back foot by rotating to the opposite side. You may rest on your elbow here and try to bring your head to the floor.

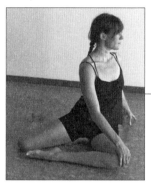 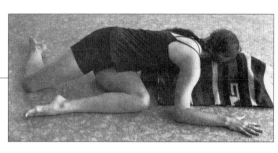

Coming Out of the Pose:

▷ Lean away from the back foot and bring that leg forward, coming back to Butterfly and ready to do the second side.

Counterposes:

▷ Since this is an external and internal hip rotation, the best counterpose is to do the other side.

▷ Windshield Wipers can be done lying down, sitting up, or reclining on the elbows.

Meridians & Organs Affected:

▷ If the front leg is firmly on the floor or if you are twisting, the Gall Bladder line is activated. Any inner groin sensations indicate that the Liver and Kidneys are benefiting. If the thigh is stretched, the Stomach and Spleen are activated.

Joints Affected:

▷ Hips mostly, but if you include the twisting version the spine will also benefit

Recommended Hold Times:

▷ Most can't do this pose well enough to get a lot of benefit from it, so it is useful mainly as a counterpose (in which case, hold for up to one minute).

Similar Yang Asanas:

▷ This is a combination of Virasana (Hero Pose) for the back leg and Padmasana (Lotus Pose) or Baddha Konasana (Butterfly) for the front leg.

Other Notes:

▷ Useful after long-held, external hip rotations such as Shoelace, Swan, or Winged Dragon.

▷ Most students won't easily understand what the pose is about . . . they won't move their feet far enough away from the groin or hips, or they will tilt too much, allowing the internally rotated hip to rise off the floor. Teachers will have to inspect the efforts of their students and offer guidance.

Dragons

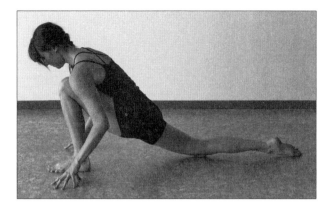

Benefits:

▷ Deep hip and groin opener that gets right into the joint

▷ Stretches the back leg's hip flexors and quadriceps

▷ Many variations to help work deeply into the hip socket

▷ Can help with sciatica

Contraindications:

▷ Can be uncomfortable for the kneecap or ankle. If you are stiff, the back thigh will be at a 90 degree angle to the front thigh, putting a lot of weight on the kneecap. Support the back knee with a blanket, or place a bolster under the shin, allowing the back knee to be off the floor.

Getting Into the Pose:

▷ Begin either on hands and knees or in Down Dog. Step one foot between the hands. Walk the front foot forward until the knee is right above the heel. Slide the back knee backward as far as you can. Keep the hands on either side of the front foot.

Alternatives & Options:

▷ If the back knee is uncomfortable, place a blanket under it, rest the shin on a bolster, or tuck the toes under and lift the leg off the floor. Lifting the back leg off the floor is much more advanced.

▷ If the ankle is uncomfortable, place a blanket underneath or raise the knee by putting a bolster under the shin.

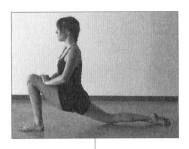

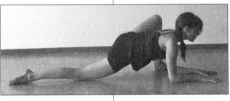

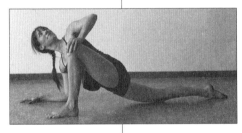

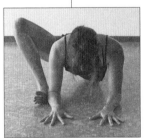

▷ Press the top of the back foot down firmly, emphasizing the little toe.

▷ The first alternative pose is a simple low lunge called Baby Dragon, as shown in the picture at the top of the previous page. If you like, you can rest your hands on blocks.

▷ The next option is to rest the arms or hands on the front thigh and lift the chest, increasing the weight over the hips. This is called Dragon Flying High.

▷ A deeper option, Dragon Flying Low, is to place both hands inside the front foot and walk hands forward, lowering the hips. For more depth, come down on the elbows or rest them on a bolster or block.

▷ In Twisted Dragon, one hand pushes the front knee to the side, while the chest rotates to the sky.

▷ In Winged Dragon, with hands on the floor, wing out the knee a few times, rolling onto the outside edge of that foot and then stay there with the knee low. You could come down on the elbows or rest them on a block or bolster.

- ▷ Overstepping Dragon exercises the ankle. From Baby Dragon, allow the front knee to come far forward and/or slide the heel backward, until the heel is just about to lift off the ground.

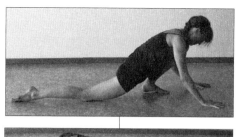

- ▷ Dragon Splits offers the deepest stretch for hip flexors. Straighten both legs into the splits. Support the front hip with a bolster under the buttock for balance and to release weight; this relaxes the muscles. Sit up tall or fold forward for different sensations.

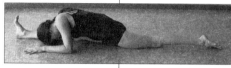

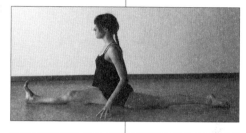

- ▷ For Fire-Breathing Dragon, in any of the above variations, tuck the back toe under and lift the knee up, lengthening the leg. This puts more weight into the hips, increasing the stretch.

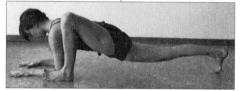

Coming Out of the Pose:

- ▷ Move your paws to Down Dog position, move the back knee forward a bit, tuck the back toes under, and with a nice groan, step back to Down Dog.

Counterposes:

- ▷ A short Down Dog is delicious. Bend one knee, lifting that heel and pushing the opposite heel down, and then switch sides repeatedly.
- ▷ Child's Pose feels really good after Down Dog and before switching to the other side of the Dragon.

Meridians & Organs Affected:

▷ Stomach, Spleen, Liver, Gall Bladder, and Kidneys (and the Urinary Bladder in Dragon Flying High or Dragon Splits High)

Joints Affected:

▷ Hips and ankles

▷ Lower back in the backbend options

Recommended Hold Times:

▷ Hold each variation for one minute and cycle through all of them.

▷ Hold just one variation for three to five minutes.

Similar Yang Asanas:

▷ Low lunge (Anjaneyasana). Sometimes this pose becomes the "Pedicure Fixing Asana" due to the urge to fix up your pedicure. At these times, allow the urge to arise but don't react to it!

Other Notes:

▷ You may not feel anything in the outer hip joint. If your hip flexors or quadriceps are tight, that area will take all the stress. This is still a good pose, but to work your hips, other poses will be needed.

Frog

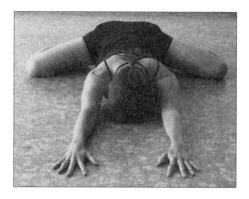

Benefits:

▷ Deep groin opener (especially the adductors)

▷ Provides a slight backbend, which compresses the lower and upper back

▷ Aids digestion and relieves cramps—both menstrual cramps and those from eating.

Contraindications:

▷ If you have a bad back.

▷ Knees can be uncomfortable, so use padding underneath.

▷ If the neck is stiff, rest the forehead, not the chin, on the floor or a bolster.

▷ If prone to tingling in the hands when you extend the arms overhead, you may need to move the hands wider apart or closer together. If that doesn't help, do one arm at a time.

Getting Into the Pose:

▷ Start in Child's Pose and slide both hands forward, separate the knees, but remain sitting on the heels. This is also known as the Tadpole.

Alternatives & Options:

▷ Half Frog: lift the hips higher, until they are in line with the knees. Keep feet together.

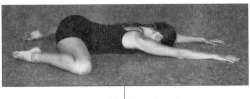

▷Full Frog: separate the feet as wide as the knees.

▷Extend one arm at a time, which is safer than extending both arms forward. The other arm can be bent with the head resting on the forearm.

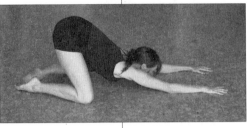

▷Allow the hips to come further forward if pressure in the groin or hips is too severe.

▷Alternately, keep toes together and allow hips to go backward.

▷May rest the chest on a bolster to relax the upper body.

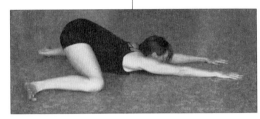

▷If the shoulders are uncomfortable, spread the hands further apart.

Coming Out of the Pose:

▷ Either sit back into Child's Pose or slide forward onto your belly, bringing your legs together.

Counterposes:

▷ Child's Pose

▷ Lying on your back, hug the knees to your chest and rock side to side or move knees in circles.

Meridians & Organs Affected:

▷ Spleen (inner knees), Liver, and Kidney (inner groins) meridians

▷ When the arms are stretched forward, the upper body meridians are massaged, affecting the meridians of Heart, Lungs, and Small and Large Intestines

Joints Affected:

▷ Hips, lower back, and shoulders

Recommended Hold Times:

▷ Three to five minutes

Similar Yang Asanas:

▷ Mandukasana or Bhekasana

Other Notes:

▷ When the hips are in line with the knees, gravity has maximum effect. Often students will move hips forward to avoid painful compression in the hips—that is okay.

▷ If doing this right after eating, rest on the elbows and don't let the stomach rest on the floor. Allow it to hang, which is nice for digestion.

▷ A nice pose to begin a class or if short of time.

▷ To advance in this posture, don't go deeper, just stay longer!

▷ You could do the first half of the pose in Tadpole and then move to Full Frog for the second half.

Happy Baby

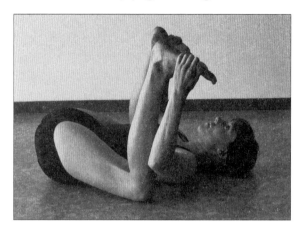

Benefits:

▷ A deep hip opener and one that can use arm strength, rather than let-ting gravity do the work

▷ If you do pull with the arms, the arm flexion strengthens the biceps.

▷ Releases and decompresses the sacroiliac (SI) joints

▷ Can be a compression of stomach organs

Contraindications:

▷ If the hips roll up off the floor, this can become a mild inversion and a mild flexion of the spine. If you have any lower back disorders which do not allow flexion of the spine, then do not allow the hips to roll off the floor.

▷ Women in their menstrual cycles may choose to also not allow their hips to roll off the floor.

▷ If there are problems in the SI joints, don't go too deep.

Getting Into the Pose:

▷ Lying on your back, hug the knees to your chest. Grab the soles of the feet, the ankles, or the back of the legs. Open the feet apart so that they are above your knees, and pull the knees towards the floor alongside your chest. Relax your head and shoulders down to the floor.

Alternatives & Options:

▷ Half Happy Baby (like an upside down Baby Dragon), holding one foot at a time.

▷ If you're very tight, you may use a belt to hold your feet, or you may do this against a wall. It is like a lying down Squat, but with the feet pushing into the wall.

▷ Can hold the backs of the thighs.

▷ Can keep your toes together for a first stage, leaving them near the groin; for a later stage, bring the toes to your nose.

▷ Eventually, feet go behind the head! (Eventually, not necessarily in this lifetime.)

▷ After a few minutes of active pulling with the arms, relax and just let the weight of the legs draw the knees down to the floor.

There are two options you can try here:

1) Allow the tailbone to curve up in the air (releases the SI joints).

2) Keep the tailbone low to the ground. Notice the differences!

A deeper option that can work the hamstrings as well as the hips is to gradually straighten the legs while still pulling the feet down and wider apart, but in this option do not allow your hips to lift off the floor.

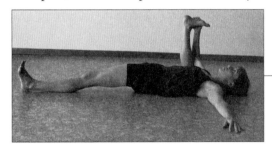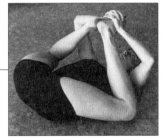

Coming Out of the Pose:

▷ Release the feet, placing them on the floor, with the knees bent. Pause for a moment.

Counterposes:

▷ Gentle backbends (lying on stomach) or, while on the back, a mild spinal lift, coming up only halfway.

▷ Windshield Wipers while lying down moves the hips from the external rotation of Happy Baby into an internal rotation. Lying down with your knees bent and your feet on the floor as wide apart as the mat, drop the knees from side to side.

Meridians & Organs Affected:

▷ Stimulates the spine and thus the Urinary Bladder, and Kidney meridians while stimulation through the inner groins also works the Liver meridians.

Joints Affected:

▷ Hips and SI/lumbar spine

Recommended Hold Times:

▷ Two minutes if you are actively pulling with the arms, but if you relax the arms, you can linger up to five minutes.

Similar Yang Asanas:

▷ Beginner's version of Yoga Nidra. Also called Window or, in Los Angeles, Dead Bug; Sarah Powers calls this Stirrup Pose.

Other Notes:

▷ This posture is the single most important reason that video recording equipment and cameras are not allowed in yoga studios.

Reclining Twist

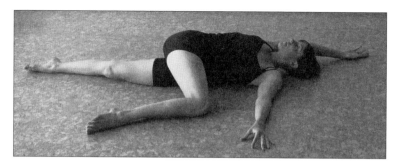

Benefits:

▷ Twisting at the end of the practice helps to restore equilibrium in the nervous system and release tension in the spine.

▷ Sarah Powers notes that bringing the bent knee more to the chest can relieve sciatica.

▷ Massages the stomach organs and cures gastritis

Contraindications:

▷ If you have shoulder issues (such as rotator cuff injuries) or are prone to tingling in the hands when you extend your arms overhead, you may not want to raise your arm to rest beside the ear or to let it float. Instead, bend the raised arm or support it with a bolster. If tingling persists, draw the hand lower or rest it on the ribs.

Getting Into the Pose:

▷ Lying on your back, draw both knees into your chest. Open your arms to the side like wings and drop the knees to one side.

Alternatives & Options:

▷ Directing the knees lower, or higher, will affect where in the spine the stretch is felt. If the knees are higher, this moves the twist to the upper back; lowering the knees moves the twist more to the lumbar/sacrum.

▷ For a deeper twist, draw one knee into the chest and, holding that knee with the opposite hand, draw it across the body. Rock back and forth a few times, but try to keep the shoulder blades flat on the floor. If the shoulder is off the floor, place a bolster under the bent knee(s).

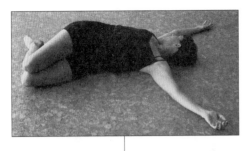

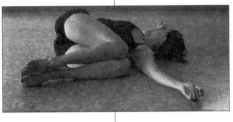

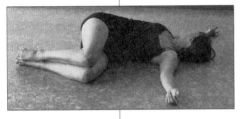

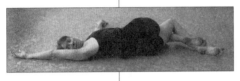

▷ If the shoulder is still floating, place a blanket under the shoulder or a bolster along the spine.

▷ Experiment with the head, turning your head to either side, and notice how the sensations change.

▷ The hand alongside the ear can be resting on the floor or on a bolster.

▷ Try the Twisted Roots pose with knees crossed as in eagle pose (Garudasana).

▷ Placing the top leg straight out to the side applies the most leverage, which helps to keep the hips fully turned. For some, it's less of a twist and more of a stretch to the outside of the leg and hip: great for the IT band. The deepest version of this option is to hold the foot with the opposite hand.

Coming Out of the Pose:

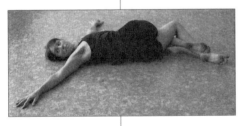

▷ Slowly roll onto your back and hug the knees into the chest to release the sacrum and lumbar.

Counterposes:

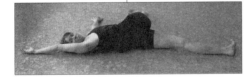

▷ Hug the knees and rock on your back from side to side.

▷ Windshield Wipers while lying back can be a nice release.

▷ Lying down with your knees bent and your feet on the floor as wide apart as the mat, drop the knees from side to side.

Meridians & Organs Affected:

▷ Twisting the spine stimulates the Urinary Bladder lines (the ida and pingala nadis).

▷ If one arm is overhead, several meridians in that arm are stimulated— the Heart, Lung, Small Intestines, and Large Intestines.

▷ Twists compress the stomach and massage the internal organs. Twisting through the rib cage stimulates the Gall Bladder meridians.

▷ Helps the liver, spleen, and pancreas[9]

Joints Affected:

▷ Nurtures the shoulder joint and upper spine, as well as all the tissues in the upper chest, breast, and shoulder.

▷ When the knee is at 90 degrees or less, the lower spine, especially the lumbar and sacroiliac joints are stressed.

Recommended Hold Time:

▷ Three to five minutes

Similar Yang Asanas:

▷ Jatharaparivartanasana

Other Notes:

▷ An excellent final pose of the practice because it removes kinks and knots

▷ You can slide right from this pose into Shavasana.

▷ If tingling occurs in the arms or hands, move them lower until the blood flows again. This is good advice for any yoga pose! Do not tolerate tingling, because this could be a sign that you are damaging a nerve.

▷ Twisted Roots is a great way to internally rotate the hips after a lot of external hip rotation work, such as Shoelace, Swan, Square or Winged Dragon poses.

▷ Don't push into the twist, relax. Let gravity do the work.

Saddle

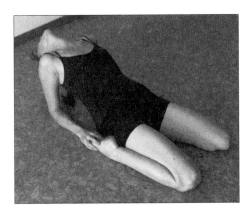

BENEFITS:

- ▷ A deep compression in the sacral-lumbar arch
- ▷ Stretches hip flexors and quadriceps
- ▷ Excellent for athletes and people who do a lot of standing or walking[10]
- ▷ Stimulates the thyroid if the neck is dropped back
- ▷ If the foot is, or the feet are, beside the hips, this becomes a good internal rotation of the hip.

CONTRAINDICATIONS:

- ▷ If you have a bad back or tight sacroiliac (SI) joints
- ▷ Knees can be tested too much here.
- ▷ Ankles can protest.
- ▷ If any sharp or burning pain here, you must come out!

GETTING INTO THE POSE:

- ▷ There are several options for coming into this pose. Start with simply sitting on the heels and notice how this feels. If there's pain in the knees, skip this one. If your ankles are complaining, try a blanket under them or skip the pose. Lean back on your hands, creating a little arch to the lower back. Check in with how this feels. This may be it for you today! If you can go further, come down onto your elbows.

Alternatives & Options:

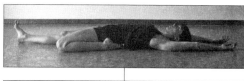

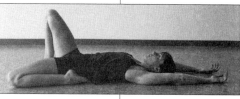

▷ If this is too deep for the lower back, do the Sphinx pose.

▷ You can also straighten one leg for Half Saddle. You can bend the straight leg and place the foot on the floor (note pictures). A deep variation is to hug the top knee toward the chest. That can get quite juicy.

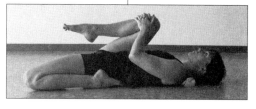

▷ If you can only go as far back as your elbows, rest on a bolster to relax here. There are various ways you may use bolsters—stack two crossways under the shoulders, or use just one, or place one lengthwise under the spine.

▷ Resting the top of the head on the floor opens the throat.

▷ Arms overhead can open the shoulders and intensify the stretch in the hip flexors.

▷ Lift the hips even higher by placing a block between the feet and under the buttocks.

▷ A blanket or rolled-up towel under the ankles can relieve pressure there.

▷ Sarah Powers often adds a twist in the Saddle by bringing a hand behind the back and grabbing the inner thigh, which stimulates the shoulder lines. In this version, you won't lean back onto the head or the elbows; from sitting, just arch back and remember to do both sides!

▷ Play with sitting on the heels and between the heels; the first emphasizes the lumbar more, and the second works the quads and hip flexors more.

Coming Out of the Pose:

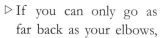

▷ There are several ways to end this pose. If you can, come back up the way you went down, propping yourself up on your elbows and then onto the hands. Lie down on your belly, straightening your legs slowly to allow the knees to release.

> If that doesn't work and you are stuck, rent a crane or a forklift. If they are not available, trying rolling to one side and slowly straighten the opposite leg. Before rolling onto your back, you may want to wait a bit or hold your sacrum with your free hand and ease down to your back.

> If you're flexible, you can just lift your knees up and pop your feet out.

Counterposes:

> After coming out, lie quietly on your back for a few breaths with the legs straight, tightening and releasing the kneecaps. When you are ready, hug the backs of the thighs and pull the knees to the chest to release the lower back.

> Child's Pose: move into it slowly. You may need to rest your head on your palms before coming into a full Child's Pose.

> Crocodile or Push-up engage the knees and tone the core of the body.

> If you came out and are lying on your back, try Hinge: while lying on your back, raise and lower the legs; knees bent is easiest, straight legs is harder. To support the back, place your hands, with palms down, under your buttocks.

Meridians & Organs Affected:

> Stomach, Spleen, Urinary Bladder, and Kidney lines

> If your arms are overhead, you will also work the Heart and Lung meridians.

Joints Affected:

> The SI joints, lower spine, knees, and ankles

Recommended Hold Times:

> One to five minutes

> Iyengar says up to 15 minutes![11]

Similar Yang Asanas:

> Supta Vajrasana or Supta Virasana

Other Notes:

▷ This is not a deep backbend for experienced yogis who are already very open in the lower back; however, this pose does work many areas at once: ankles, knees, quadriceps, hip flexors, sacrum and lumbar, and shoulders.

▷ Can be done right after eating.

▷ If your job requires you to stand all day and you do this pose at night before bed, your legs will feel rested in the morning.

▷ Unlike the yang poses, don't tuck the tailbone as we normally would in backbends.

Shoelace

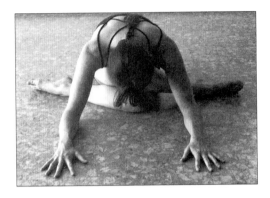

Benefits:

▷ A great hip opener and decompression for the lower spine when folding forward

Contraindications:

▷ Hard on the pelvis and knees and can aggravate sciatica. If you have sciatica, elevate the hips by sitting on a cushion so the knees are below them. Beware of hips rotating backward while seated; we want them to rotate forward.

▷ If you have any lower back disorders which do not allow flexion of the spine, then do not allow the spine to round: keep the back as straight as you can.

▷ Pregnant women should not fold forward after the first trimester.

Getting Into the Pose:

▷ There are several options for coming into this pose. One way is to begin by kneeling on all fours, then place one knee behind the other and sit back between the heels. A second approach is to begin by sitting on your heels and then slide onto one buttock and bring the outside foot over toward the opposite hip. A third approach is to begin by sitting cross-legged and then draw one foot under the opposite thigh and the other foot over toward the opposite hip.

▷ Try not to sit on the feet but slide them as far forward as they can go. Anchor both sitting bones to the ground.

Alternatives & Options:

▷ If hips are tight, sit on a bolster to tilt them forward.

▷ If the bottom knee complains, do the pose with the bottom leg straight. If the top knee complains, place a bolster or blanket under that knee. If this is still too hard, sit cross-legged and fold forward.

▷ Support the chest with bolster.

▷ When folding forward, you can support the head with the hands, leaning the elbows onto the thighs or a block or bolster.

▷ Hands can be to the side or in front of the body, or stretch the arms back behind the body.

▷ If sensations are too intense in the hips or knees, remain upright or take more weight into the hands and arms.

▷ Sidebends or twists can be added here, which work the Gall Bladder meridian.

▷ Other alternatives include Eye-of-the-Needle Pose (lying on your back, cradle your shin in your arms), Square Pose, or Swan.

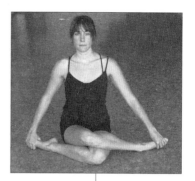

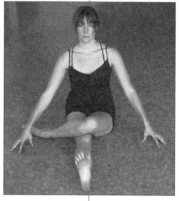

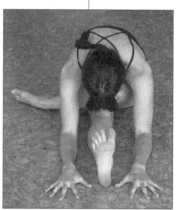

Coming Out of the Pose:

▷ Lean back to release the hips and slowly straighten the legs.

Counterposes:

▷ Windshield Wipers lying down or sitting (to provide an internal rotation of the hip)

▷ Deer Pose

▷ Tabletop (aka Hammock)

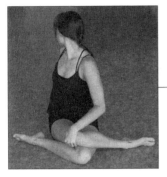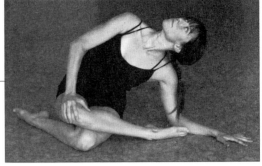

Meridians & Organs Affected:

▷ Liver, Kidney, and Gall Bladder. If folding forward, the Urinary Bladder line will be stimulated and the stomach compressed.

Joints Affected:

▷ Hips and lower spine

Recommended Hold Times:

▷ Three to five minutes per side

Similar Yang Asanas:

▷ Cowface (Gomukasana)

Other Notes:

▷ It is nice to follow this with Swan or Sleeping Swan before doing the other side.

▷ Could do a sitting twist afterward.

▷ Start with the more-open hip first (whichever hip is more open, place that knee on top).

▷ Keep weight back into sitting bones when you come forward, preventing the weight from moving into the knees.

▷ Keep hips even. There is a tendency for the top hip to be pulled forward.

▷ While you are lingering in this pose, try some poses targeting the shoulders or wrists. Check the section on the upper body for some suggestions.

▷ You could do the first half of the time in a variation like sidebend or twist and then fold forward for the remaining time.

Snail

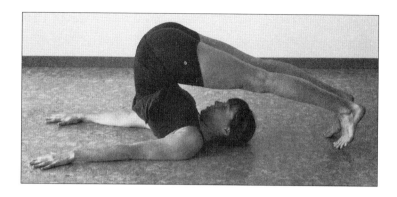

Benefits:

▷ One of the deepest releases of the whole spine

▷ Relaxes the heart, brings more blood flow to the head, drains the lungs, and compresses the internal organs, giving them a great massage

Contraindications:

▷ This pose puts a lot of pressure on the neck; be cautious! Avoid if you have any neck problems.

▷ Not recommended for anyone with high blood pressure, upper body infection, vertigo, glaucoma, or a cold; also women who are menstruating may find it better not to do this pose.

▷ If you have any lower back disorders which do not allow flexion of the spine, then do not attempt this posture.

▷ Do not do this posture if you have recently eaten or are pregnant.

Getting Into the Pose:

▷ Start in a lying down position. Lift your hips and support them with your hands. Allow your back to round (unlike the Plough pose, Halasana, in which we strive to keep the spine and legs straight) and your feet to fall over your head toward the floor. Position the weight of your body onto your shoulders; note how much weight is on your neck—some is okay, but not too much!

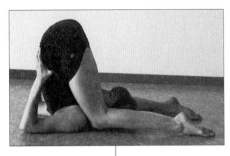

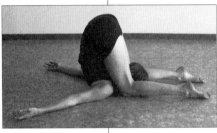

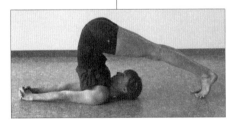

Alternatives & Options:

▷There are many intermediate stages to this pose. For beginners, or those not wishing to invert, replace this pose with a seated, straight leg, forward fold (such as Caterpillar).

▷There are three stages to the posture:

1) Support the back with the palms.

2) More challenging (but not shown) is to place palms under the feet and lower the feet to the floor, or rest them on a bolster.

3) Most challenging is to bend the knees toward the floor (the deepest rounding for the spine).

▷Very challenging option: with the knees bent toward the floor, twist until both knees are on one side of the head. Remember to do both sides.

▷ If legs are straight and feet are touching the floor, the hands can come to the floor behind the back. Hands can be apart (easier) or together (if there are no shoulder problems), but be careful; bringing the hands together could aggravate rotator cuff problems.

Coming Out of the Pose:

▷ The simplest way to come out is to keep the knees bent and hold your hips. Allow yourself to slowly roll down. Your head will likely lift up as you come down. Don't strain to keep your head on the floor.

▷ More challenging is to come out with the legs straight and holding the feet. Slowly roll down, holding the feet as a way to slow your descent.

Counterposes:

▷ After coming out, lie down for a few breaths with the knees bent and feet flat on the floor.

▷ Do Windshield Wipers then a gentle backbend, such as lying on the stomach, or a mild spinal lift. Come up only halfway.

▷ Gentle Fish (Matsyasana) helps to release the neck and move the spine into extension.

▷ If Fish pose is too much, if the neck feels weak or tweaked, do an Upward Facing Cat instead.

▷ Child's Pose.

Meridians & Organs Affected:

▷ All internal organs are massaged and compressed, and each breath adds to the massage.

▷ Urinary Bladder lines are deeply stretched.

Joints Affected:

▷ The full spine

Recommended Hold Times:

▷ Three to five minutes

Similar Yang Asanas:

▷ Halasana (Plough) or Karnapidasana (Resting Pose or Ear Pressure Pose)

Other Notes:

▷ Prepare the neck first by doing gentle forward neck bends.

▷ A nice alternative is Happy Baby, which allows the sacrum to lift off the floor.

▷ Allow the spine to fully round. Do not try to keep the spine straight and the hips high.

Sphinx & Seal

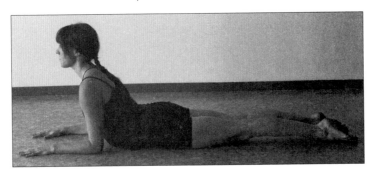

Benefits:

> ▷ Can be a very deep compression and stimulation of the sacral-lumbar arch. Between the L2 and L3 vertebrae is found the "Door of Life," where Jing energy is housed.

> ▷ Tones the spine. People with bulging or herniated disks may find this very therapeutic.[12]

> ▷ If the neck is dropped back, the thyroid will also be stimulated.

> ▷ In the full Seal pose, the stomach may receive a lovely stretch, as well.

Contraindications:

> ▷ If you have a bad back or tight sacrum.

> ▷ If there are any sharp pains here, you must come out!

> ▷ Avoid pressing the belly into the floor if you're pregnant (use bolsters under the pelvis and the forearms).

> ▷ Avoid if you have a headache.

Getting Into the Pose:

> ▷ Lie down on your belly. Clasp your elbows with the opposite hands and move the elbows just ahead of your shoulders, propping yourself up. Notice how this feels in your lower back. If the sensations are too strong, move your elbows further ahead, lowering your chest closer to the floor. If you like, you can place your palms flat on the floor in front of you like a sphinx.

Alternatives & Options:

▷ For a gentle Sphinx, rest on the ribs, sliding the elbows away to reduce compression in the lower back. Simply lying on your stomach may be enough of a backbend for you.

▷ You can use a cushion under the elbows, helping to elevate the chest and deepen the posture.

▷ Alternatively, you can place a bolster under the arm pits and relax completely.

▷ Seal pose with straight, locked arms is the deepest pose; let the hands rotate outward a little. Slide your hands away to lessen the intensity.

▷ You may feel the highest amount of compression in the lower back if your hands are not right under the shoulders but slightly forward. This provides some pressure in the lower back.

▷ Rather than have the arms in front, Paulie Zink likes to have the hands and arms straight out to the side, which makes this look more like a seal.

▷ Bend the knees for more compression in the sacrum.

▷ You may spread the legs apart to deepen the sensations in the lower back.

▷ You may prefer to keep the legs together to release the sacrum or make the sensations more even along the spine.

▷ You can place a bolster or blanket under the pubic bone or thighs to soften the pressure. This is really nice for pregnant women.

▷ Tightening the buttocks is okay within reason. Sagging the shoulders is also okay.

▷ To arch the neck and stimulate the cervical spine, lengthen the neck, drop the head back, lift the chin, and open the throat.

▷ If your head gets too heavy for your neck, try resting your head in your hands or your chin on your fists.

▷ If you're flexible, try these postures with the legs in lotus.

COMING OUT OF THE POSE:

▷ To come out, slowly lower your chest to the floor. Turn your head to one side and rest your cheek on your palms. You may wish to decompress the lower back more by sliding one knee up. Choose the knee that you are looking toward, and keep the knee and foot on the floor.

COUNTERPOSES:

▷ Child's Pose is a nice, gentle forward fold; move into it slowly. You may need to rest your head on your palms.

▷ On your way to Child's Pose you may crave Cat's Breath: flow from the Upward Facing Cat to the Downward Facing Cat (aka Cat/Cow) but flow gently, in time with the breath. Don't make these your deepest Cats ever.

MERIDIANS & ORGANS AFFECTED:

▷ Urinary Bladder and Kidney lines, as well as the Stomach and Spleen meridians

▷ Stimulates the kidneys and adrenal glands through compression[13]

JOINTS AFFECTED:

▷ Lower spine and the neck (if dropped back)

RECOMMENDED HOLD TIMES:

▷ Sphinx can be held longer than Seal.

▷ For Seal, start with one-minute holds, then lower down, rest, and repeat several times.

▷ Up to five minutes

▷ Eventually up to twenty minutes!

SIMILAR YANG ASANAS:

▷ Sphinx and/or Cobra

OTHER NOTES:

▷ Imagine the spine like a row of Christmas tree lights draping to the floor.

▷ If the arms are straight, this pose is a deeper backbend than Saddle and, thus, could be done after Saddle. If the arms are bent (as in Sphinx), this is not as deep as Saddle, so it may be done beforehand.

▷ Seal is nice and safe if you're pregnant.

▷ Ideal for adding some breath work and conscious energy movement

▷ Great pose for watching television!

Square

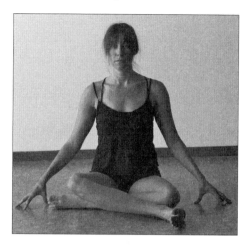

Benefits:

    ▷ Nice preparation for Lotus Pose

    ▷ A deep opening of the hips through strong external rotation

    ▷ Decompresses the lower back when folding forward

Contraindications:

    ▷ Watch the pressure on the knees; if the hips are too tight, the pressure will go there.

    ▷ Can aggravate sciatica. If you have sciatica, elevate the hips by sitting on a cushion, until the knees are below the hips, or avoid this pose entirely. Beware of hips rotating backward while seated; we want them to rotate forward.

    ▷ If you have any lower back disorders which do not allow flexion of the spine, then do not allow the spine to round: keep the back as straight as you can.

Getting Into the Pose:

    ▷ This can be a tricky one to get into. The key is to go where you feel some juiciness in the outer hips, never in the knees. Start by sitting with legs crossed. Move your feet forward until your shins are parallel to the front edge of your mat (your legs are "square" to it).

    ▷ Try to move your knees closer together without allowing your feet to come back closer to you.

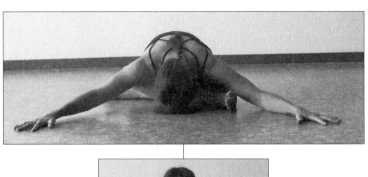

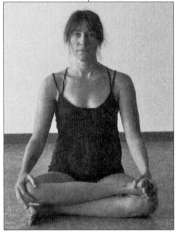

Alternatives & Options:

▷ Folding forward stretches the lower back and can intensify the stress in the hips. If you can't come forward, sit on a cushion.

▷ A deeper option is to place one ankle over the opposite knee and the other ankle under its opposite knee. If the first knee is very high in the air, you are not ready for this variation! Bring that foot to the floor in front of its opposite knee.

▷ If you're more flexible, try to slide the knees closer together, allowing the feet go further apart.

▷ If you're tight or experience discomfort in the knees, or if the knees are high off the floor, you can place blankets or some form of support under the knees.

▷ Other alternatives include Eye-of-the-Needle Pose, Shoelace, or Swan.

Coming Out of the Pose:

▷ Lean back and slowly straighten the legs out in front of you.

Counterposes:

▷ Bounce out the legs and tighten/release the knees a few times.

▷ This was a fairly deep external rotation of the hips, so we want to move the hips in the opposite direction. Some nice internal rotations of the hips are Deer or Windshield Wipers.

▷ If you're craving a backbend, perform Tabletop or lie down and do some Spinal Lifts.

Meridians & Organs Affected:

▷ Liver, Kidneys, and Gall Bladder

▷ Urinary Bladder line (if folding forward)

Joints Affected:

▷ Hips and spine

Recommended Hold Times:

▷ Three to five minutes per side

Similar Yang Asanas:

▷ Double Pigeon (sometimes called Boxcar, 90-90, or Fire Logs)

Other Notes:

▷ If you're a beginner, you may tend to bring your feet close to the groin. Make sure this isn't simply a cross-legged sitting posture; we want to feel this in the hips.

▷ However, if you already feel this is stressing the hips a lot, simply by sitting cross-legged, then that is your version of Square pose! Be there and enjoy.

Squat

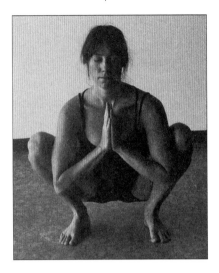

Benefits:

   ▷ Opens the hips and strengthens the ankles

   ▷ Releases the lower back

   ▷ Can be a great pose to prepare the body for childbirth

   ▷ Offers relief to women suffering severe lower back pain due to their menstrual cycle[14]

Contraindications:

   ▷ If hips are too tight, this can torque the knees.

   ▷ If you have knee trauma, avoid this pose.

Getting Into the Pose:

   ▷ Start by standing with the feet hip-width apart. Squat down and bring your arms in front of you, hands in prayer and elbows pulling lightly against the knees or shins.

Alternatives & Options:

   ▷ If your heels are off the floor, use a folded blanket or bolster under them. We want the body to relax. Another option if the heels are off the floor is to widen the distance between the feet.

▷ Watch where the knees are pointing compared to where the feet are pointing. They should point in the same direction. If they are not, spread the feet wider or rest the heels on a folded blanket or on a bolster.

▷ When the feet are wide apart (hip width or more), this pose works into the hips more deeply.

▷ When the feet are close together (perhaps even touching), this pose works the ankles more deeply.

▷ A deep variation is to keep the feet together but with the knees wide apart. Lean forward, wrapping your arms around the shins and then behind the back, clasping the hands together.

▷ Another option is to place your hands behind your head and gently draw the chin to the chest: this adds a stretch to the back of the neck.

Coming Out of the Pose:

▷ An easy exit is to just sit down and then slowly straighten the legs out in front of you.

▷ A more challenging exit is to come to Dangling by straightening the legs and folding forward. As you straighten the legs, align the feet so that they are pointing in the same direction as your knees.

Counterposes:

▷ Dangling, as just described, helps to release the knees and back.

▷ Ankle stretch or Vajrasana. In Vajrasana, keep the knees together and sit on the heels.

Meridians & Organs Affected:

▷ The Liver, Kidney, and Urinary Bladder lines

▷ If you feel this through your ankles you may also be stimulating the Stomach, Spleen, Gall Bladder, and Urinary Bladder meridians.

Joints Affected:

▷ Hips, knees, and ankles

Recommended Hold Times

▷ Two to three minutes at one time; however, you can revisit this pose a couple of times during the practice.

Similar Yang Asanas:

▷ Malasana

Other Notes:

▷ Approximately two-thirds of the world's population goes to the bath-room every day this way! If uncomfortable, it may be a sign that you need to do this more.

▷ A nice sequence is to go from Dangling to Squat, back to Dangling, back to Squat, over and over again, holding each position for one to two minutes.

▷ Elbows in front of knees can be used as levers to pull the chest forward, allowing the tailbone to drop lower.

Straddle (Dragonfly)

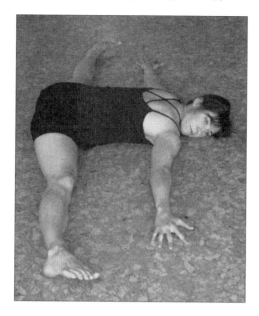

Benefits:

▷ Opens the hips, groin, and the backs of the thighs

▷ Provides a gentle opening to the inner knees

▷ Stimulates the ovaries

Contraindications:

▷ Can aggravate sciatica. If you have this condition, elevate the hips. Beware of hips rotating backward while seated; we want them to rotate forward.

▷ If you have any lower back disorders which do not allow flexion of the spine, then do not allow the spine to round: keep the back as straight as you can.

▷ If you have any inner knee trauma or issues, bring the legs closer together or tighten the top of the legs (the quadriceps) to engage the kneecaps.

Getting Into the Pose:

▷ From a sitting position, spread your legs apart until they won't go any further. Sitting on a cushion will help tilt your hips. Fold forward, resting your weight into your hands with your arms locked straight, or rest your elbows onto a block.

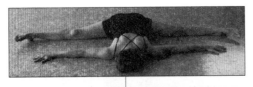

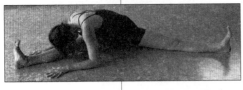

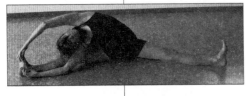

Alternatives & Options:

▷Use a bolster to raise the hips.

▷Can keep hands behind the back.

▷Folding over one leg increases spinal and hamstring stretch.

▷If the knees feel bothered, tighten the quadriceps to close the knee joint or bring legs closer together.

▷If hamstrings feel too tight, bend the knee(s) and place a bolster under the thigh(s).

▷Legs can be 90 degrees apart to 120 degrees for advanced students. The full split of 180 degrees is not necessary, but if you can do it, go for it.

▷If you're advanced, fold right down onto your stomach and rest your arms to the sides.

▷Use a bolster under the chest, if you are close to the floor.

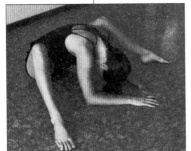

▷ If your head is too heavy for your neck, support it in your hands.

▷ If you are stiff, bend the knees a lot! It is also okay to place the feet flat on the floor. When the knees are bent, and while sitting on a cushion, you can bend forward more easily and allow gravity to do the work.

▷ Can come into a twist by folding over one leg and rotating chest skyward (if advanced, hold the foot with both hands)

▷ Can also do a sitting up twist (which helps to stimulate the upper body meridians under the scapula).

Coming Out of the Pose:

▷ Use your hands to push the floor away and slowly roll up.

▷ Once you are up, lean back on your hands to release the hips, tighten the leg muscles, and drag or lift your legs to bring them together. Bounce or shake out the legs. Groaning is allowed. (Groans coming out of Yin Yoga poses sound like "ommmm." Om is the first syllable of "OhmiGod!")

Counterposes:

▷ Windshield Wipers are nice, or do a cross-legged, seated backbend.

▷ Tabletop (aka Hammock)

Meridians & Organs Affected:

▷ Urinary Bladder, Liver, Kidney, and Spleen

▷ The twisting version will stimulate the Gall Bladder.

Joints Affected:

▷ Hips, lower back, and knees

Recommended Hold Times:

▷ Three to ten minutes

Similar Yang Asanas:

▷ Upavistakonasana

Other Notes:

▷ Very frustrating for beginners: the adductor muscles tug on the sitting bones, just like the hamstrings do, which causes the top of the hips to tilt backward. Persistence is required! Sitting on a bolster helps.

▷ Keep weight forward on the sitting bones; even tug the flesh away from the buttocks before folding forward.

▷ Often it is nice to spend half of the time in one variation and then add a twist for the last half of the pose.

Swan & Sleeping Swan

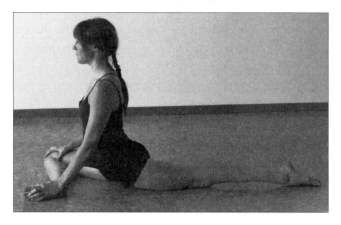

Benefits:

> ▷ A vigorous way to open the hips, allowing gravity to do the work
> ▷ Strong external rotation of front hip (especially in the image shown)
> ▷ Provides the quadriceps and hip flexors a nice stretch for the side that has the leg back
> ▷ A moderate to strong backbend, compressing the lower back
> ▷ Can control sexual desires due to lots of blood flowing through the pubic region[15]

Contraindications:

> ▷ If you have bad knees (especially any problems with the inner meniscus), watch the pressure.
> ▷ If hips are too tight, that is where the pressure will go. If this happens, bring the front foot back, more toward or under that hip.

Getting Into the Pose:

> ▷ You can come into this pose either from Down Dog (which is more advanced) or from Cat pose (on hands and knees). Slide your right knee between your hands, lean a bit to the right, and check in with how your right knee is going to feel. If the knee is fine, flex the right foot and move it forward; if the knee feels stressed, bring the foot closer in toward the right hip. Now, center yourself so your weight is even. Try tucking the back toes under and sliding the back knee away. Do this a few times until your right buttock is on the floor or as low as it is going to get.

Alternatives & Options (Swan):

▷ To protect the front knee, keep the front foot flexed.

▷ Move the hands closer to the hips to increase the weight over the front hip.

▷ If you are leaning to the bent leg side, place a support, like a folded blanket, under the bent knee's hip to center yourself.

▷ If you're really flexible, try to bring your front foot forward, parallel to the front of your mat, and slide the bent knee more to the side. Bring the foot beneath the sternum if possible.

▷ To increase the effect of gravity, tuck the back toes under and lift the knee off the floor, pulling the heel backward.

Alternatives & Options (Sleeping Swan):

▷ To protect the front knee, keep the foot flexed before coming forward.

▷ Keep the weight back into the hips as you lower yourself.

▷ Stay on the hands with the arms straight, or come on to the elbows.

▷ You could lie on a bolster placed lengthwise under the chest.

▷ If you're really flexible, try to bring the front foot forward, pull the bent knee more to the side, and lay your chest on top of the shin.

▷ Other alternatives include Eye-of-the-Needle (can be done lying down, while sitting, or with one leg against the wall), Shoelace, or Square Pose.

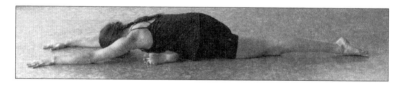

Coming Out of the Pose:

▷ Use your hands to push the floor away and slowly come up. Tuck the back toes under, plant your front paws in Down Dog position, and with a nice groan, step back to the Downward Facing Puppy. If you never liked Down Dog before, you will love it now!

Counterposes:

▷ Windshield Wipers (sitting or lying down) are a nice way to internally rotate your hips.

▷ Child's Pose (nice if you did full Swan)

▷ A Quick Down Dog before Child's Pose

Meridians & Organs Affected:

▷ Liver, Kidney, Stomach, Spleen, Gall Bladder, and the Urinary Bladder line

Joints Affected:

▷ Hips and lower back. Make sure the knees are NOT complaining!

Recommended Hold Times:

▷ This is a moderately yang posture when the chest is raised: hold one to three minutes. After a couple of minutes, switch to Sleeping Swan for another one to three minutes.

Similar Yang Asanas:

▷ Proud Pigeon (Rajakapotasana)

Other Notes:

▷ Come into full Swan from Sleeping Swan by walking the hands back toward the hips.

▷ Full Swan is a deeper hip opener than Sleeping Swan because more weight is placed right above the front hip.

▷ Full Swan can be a gentle backbend, but it can be deepened if you're really flexible by raising the arms overhead or clasping the hands behind the lower back and pulling them toward the floor.

▷ Screaming Pigeon is really a yang pose, but it can be tried at the end because those muscles won't interfere with the joints being targeted. Bend the back leg, reach the hand on the same side to that heel, and pull the heel to the buttocks. (Or until the screaming starts.)

▷ If you are feeling it, you are doing it! If you have lost the feeling, wiggle around until you find it again. Sometimes a subtle adjustment of the legs can increase the sensation in the front hip but reduce the stretch in the quadriceps of the back leg. You can decide where your priority is today.

Toe Squat

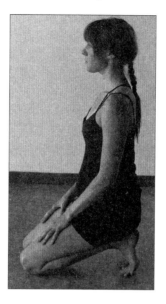

Benefits:

 ▷ Opens the toes and feet and strengthens the ankles. (Our feet are the furthest things from our minds, literally! Most of us imprison our toes all day long in shoes, and then when we are in our 70s and 80s our toes stop working and we fall down. There is an old Daoist saying; "A person with open toes has an open mind." Open your toes now!)

 ▷ Stimulates all six lines of the lower body meridians (which begin or end in the toes)

Contraindications:

 ▷ Sitting on the heels may strain the knees.

 ▷ If ankles or toe joints are very tight, don't stay here long.

Getting Into the Pose:

 ▷ Begin by sitting on your heels with the feet together. Tuck the toes under and try to be on the balls of the feet, not the tippy-toes. Reach down and tuck the little toes under.

Alternatives & Options:

 ▷ If the pose becomes too challenging, stand up on the knees, relieving most of the pressure on the toe joints. When you feel you can handle it again, sit back down on the heels.

▷ Don't stay if in pain!

▷ You can combine this posture with shoulder exercises like Eagle arms or Cow Face arms.

▷ If the knees are uncomfortable, place a blanket under them or a cushion between the hips and heels. You may enjoy a rolled-up towel behind the knees, which helps to release the knee joint.

Coming Out of the Pose:

▷ This one can be quite juicy, so come out slowly, enjoying every single minute! Lean forward onto your hands, lift your hips forward, and release your feet. Point the feet backwards and sit on your heels again. Sigh!

Counterposes:

▷ Ankle Stretch, Child's Pose, or any posture that opens the ankles, such as Saddle

Meridians & Organs Affected:

▷ All the meridians of the lower body get stimulated through the compression in the toes.

▷ The front of the ankle also becomes compressed, helping to open the Spleen, Liver, Stomach, and Gall Bladder lines.

Joints Affected:

▷ Toes and ankles

Recommended Hold Times:

▷ Two to three minutes

Similar Yang Asanas:

▷ Seiza or Vajrasana, but with the toes tucked under

Other Notes:

▷ This pose can become quite intense for most people fairly quickly. Monitor the level of intensity. It is better not to stay in the pose if you are in pain.

▷ If doing shoulder work while holding the pose, take a break between sides. Do an Ankle Stretch, and then come back into Toe Stretch and resume the shoulder work on the other side.

Shavasana

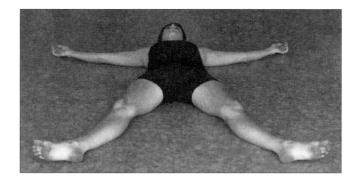

Time to relax—time to rest the body so that the body becomes stronger and healthier. Time for the little death of *Shavasana* (which literally means the "dead posture"). Shavasana symbolizes the end of your practice—a natural completion to the journey you have been on.

If you are practicing on your own, you may want to set a timer for your Shavasana. It is not uncommon for students to fall asleep. Falling asleep is okay, but most teachers prefer that you remain alert and aware while the body is relaxed. A timer will help rouse you at the end of the Shavasana. Decide how much time you need to relax. For an active yang practice, a good rule of thumb is to allow yourself 10% to 15% of your practice time. For the yin style, since the muscles were not used, a shorter period is okay—maybe 5% or 8% will suffice. However, check in with your inner guide and see how much time would be right today.

Shavasana is not just a time to relax the body; in this quiet time the mind should remain alert, yet relaxed and aware of the body relaxing. Pay attention to the energies flowing. This is an ideal time to develop your ability to feel your energies. It is difficult to do this when you are in the postures. Practicing watching the energies during your Shavasana will assist you to feel energy flowing at other times. As you actively relax, watch the flow of Chi or prana into and out of the areas you worked in the asana practice. At first you may have to pretend, or imagine, you can feel these energies. Pretending will help you look closely at these areas. In time, you will notice the energy flow more easily.

There are many ways to perform Shavasana, and many teachers have their own unique and favorite methods. Collect several ways of relaxing by taking classes with several teachers. With a larger repertoire, you can choose which way is best for any given day. The following suggestion is just one of the many possible options.

Preparing to Relax

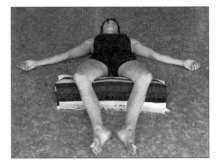

In a yoga studio, your teacher will make sure the surroundings are suitable for relaxation. If you are practicing by yourself, make your environment quiet: disconnect phones; turn off noises; open the windows to allow fresh air in, but stay warm; put any pets into another room; turn lights down, but not off completely—a completely dark room may encourage you to sleep—for the same reason you may want to avoid doing Shavasana in bed.

Begin by letting the body become open: take off glasses and watches; let your hair down; remove anything that may constrict the flow of energy. Also remove any metallic circles you have on—things like rings, bracelets, and body piercings can interfere with the flow of energy. Ensure you will stay warm—put on socks, a sweater, and/or cover yourself with a blanket. If you are doing Shavasana after a sweaty yang practice, you may need to change your shirt to avoid getting too cold, but don't wipe off any sweat; allowing sweat to dry on the body is one of the yogic healing techniques.

Make yourself comfortable as you lie down on the floor. Bending the knees a little will allow the lower back to release to the floor. If you do bend the knees, place a folded blanket or bolster under them so that the legs can relax. Allow the feet to fall inward or outward, whichever feels more relaxed. If you do not have the knees bent, separate the legs until the knees are hip-width apart or even farther. To really allow the sacrum to lie flat, slide your tailbone away from you. Next, let your arms lie beside you, palms face up and about a foot away from your hips. This will allow your shoulder blades to lie flat; snuggle them into the floor.

Lengthen the neck slightly by pointing the chin toward your feet. You can even roll your head from side to side a few times, until you find a comfortable position in the center. A pillow is nice.

Get all of your fidgeting over with: become still. Often, one or two deep breaths here with a loud sigh are delicious. Release your bones, let go completely—you are ready. Now close your eyes; time to relax.

Relax Completely

Scan your body slowly. Start with your toes and feet—allow your feet to relax. Feel them becoming heavy on the floor. Allow your awareness to rise up to the ankles, calves, and shins. Feel them melting into the earth; no effort is needed. Feel the space in the knee joints. Move slowly higher. Relax the thighs. Feel them become heavy, warm, soft. Notice your buttocks, hips, and groin relaxing; they too become soft and warm. If you have done a lot of hip work in your practice, linger here for a while feeling the openness, the flow of energy through the hips.

Now allow your awareness to come to the tailbone; feel your sacrum and lower back release into the floor. Feel your lower back and stomach muscles relax. Allow this sensation to rise up the spine. Feel each vertebra—the space between them and their alignment. Allow the upper back muscles and the shoulder blades to sink into the floor. Relax your chest and all the muscles between the ribs. Come now to the shoulders, where we carry so much tension in our bodies. Let the shoulders release completely. Spend an extra moment here, and really soften. Feel the weight of the shoulders sink into the earth. Allow this sensation of softness to flow down the arms. Relax the upper arms, the elbow, and the forearms. Feel the space in the wrist joints. Feel the space around each finger and the energy in the palm of each hand.

Bring your awareness to your neck and throat, and release all tension there. Relax your jaw, lips, and tongue; relax your cheeks and eyes and all the muscles around the eyes and deep in the eye sockets; relax your forehead and your scalp. Allow your head to rest heavily on the floor.

Now relax your inner organs. Bring your awareness to the reproductive organs, and either feel or imagine them relaxing. Relax your prostate (if you have one), intestines, and kidneys. Imagine your liver, stomach, and spleen being filled with healing energies. Soften your diaphragm and lungs. Relax your heart. Let your heart become open ... vast ... undefended, and ... smiling.

Release the breath totally: let it be whatever it wants to be. Notice the breath—become aware of the short pauses between each breath. Relax your mind ... notice that the moment between each breath is the moment between thoughts. Enjoy those moments of complete silence and peace; feel this sense of peace growing deeper. Let this feeling of peace fill you; let it fill the space around you; let peace fill the room and beyond, touching everyone and everything.

Coming Out

When the time has come, the teacher is calling you, or your timer has beckoned, begin to return to life by allowing your breath to be deeper, longer. Bring some movement to your fingers and toes while you roll your head from side to side. Take a moment to move your wrists and ankles in circles: circle in both directions to stimulate energy flow again. (There is an old Daoist saying that if you roll your ankles in circles every day, you will never die of a heart attack.) When you are ready, hug your knees to your chest in preparation for making the body small and round. Take a deep inhalation, and on the exhalation bring your head and knees together, and squeeze. Make yourself as small and as round as you can—as small as a ten-pound turkey. Release.

Wake up by stretching out the whole body—this is a natural energizer, one that many people have forgotten to do when they wake up in the morning. Move any supports away, stretch your legs along the floor and stretch your arms over your head. Interlock your fingers and turn the palms away from you. Press your lower back down; flex your toes toward your nose. Now take a huge inhalation, fill your lungs—and stretch. Make yourself as long as possible: contract all your facial muscles, and make your face as small as possible. Push and pull yourself longer. Then release with a loud sighing "haaah."

Once more, flex the toes, flatten your lower back, and take a big inhalation. Stretch your body. This time, open your face, mouth, and eyes, as wide as you can; stick your tongue out; touch your chin—stretch! Reach! Exhale, and relax with a sigh.

Hug your knees once more into your chest, and roll to your left side; pause there a moment, and let the energy settle. Stretch out your bottom arm under your head, and use it as a pillow: enjoy how this feels. Often teachers will ask students to end the class by lying on their right side to relax the heart. This is a great suggestion for ending a yang class. Lying on the right side helps to open the left nostril, due to a sinus reflex. However, the left nostril is the yin channel. After ninety minutes or so of yin practice, it is nice to balance the body by lying on the left side, allowing the right nostril, the yang channel, to open.

Don't linger too long here; coming back to life is like being reincarnated. Don't stay in the bardo state between Shavasana (your little death) and rebirth too long, or you may decide to stay there forever. When you are ready, spiral up to sitting and prepare for your final meditation or pranayama practice. If you still feel that you are not quite back to normal, you may want to end your practice with Nadi Shodhana breathing to fully balance your energies.[16]

Adverse Reactions to Shavasana—A Warning!

Several studies of the relaxation response have shown that, occasionally, relaxation can have adverse effects. These effects range from a feeling of being dissociated from your body or from reality, to feelings of anxiety or panic. Sometimes deeply repressed emotions start to surface. If these start to trouble you, remain calm, and resolve to watch whatever unfolds with the same dispassion with which you were watching the breath during your practice. If conditions persist, seek assistance.

For some students, physiological reactions can occur; blood pressure can drop after deep relaxation, and a temporary hypoglycemic state can occur. If you are on medication, deep relaxation may intensify the effect of the drugs. Caution is advised for students taking insulin, sedatives, or cardiovascular medications. Check with your health care professional before beginning a yoga practice if you are on medication.

These occurrences are rare, but it is good to be aware that adverse reactions can happen. Don't be alarmed. If the situation warrants help, seek it.

Yin Yoga Poses for the Upper Body

The practice of Yin Yoga involves stressing the yin tissues of the body safely (which means no pain), for long periods of time while staying relaxed. Note that this definition does not specify where the tissues must be. We know that the yin tissues that we are targeting are the denser, deeper, more plastic/less elastic tissues, such as the ligaments, joint capsules, cartilage, bones and fascial networks of the body, but these tissues are found in the upper body as well as the lower body. We can apply the principles of Yin Yoga all over the body, though so far have focused on the lower body because as we age it is this area that tightens up the most. From the navel down, as we get older our mobility decreases and injuries and pathologies increase. But we can, indeed, do Yin Yoga for the shoulders, neck, and arms. This section offers a few ways we can work these specific areas.

The Neck

We carry a lot of stress in the neck and shoulder area, especially when we spend great swaths of time typing or working with our hands. Tight neck and shoulder muscles can lead to headaches and shallow breathing. Chronically tight necks can lead to shortened ligaments and a very restricted range of motion. A very common movement pattern can be seen in the elderly: if you call a young child's name from behind her, she may just turn her head to look at you. As an adult, she may have to turn her whole torso, from the hips. If you call an elderly person from behind, he will likely turn his whole body, moving his feet, in order to look at you. There is an old yoga saying, "You are only as young as your spine!"

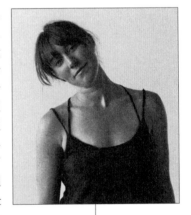

We can work the neck in six main directions while sitting in several different Yin Yoga postures. In fact most of the poses offered for the upper body can be done while sitting in Shoelace, Square, Straddle, Toe

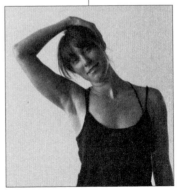

Squat, or while sitting with the legs comfortably crossed. Try the poses listed below while in the basic Shoelace position. If you have any neck issues, don't try these until you have checked with your health care provider.

Lateral (Side) Flexion

Sit on a cushion in the Shoelace posture. Keep the spine nice and long, including the neck. Drop your right ear to the right shoulder. The three principles of the practice still apply: find a nice edge so that you feel some stress on the side of the neck away from the shoulder you are leaning towards. Become still, and stay for one or two minutes. Work up to longer stays over time. If the edge moves, allow your ear to drop lower. Be cautious that you are not simply tilting your whole body, or worse, collapsing your spine. Keep sitting tall. If you would like a bit more stress, gently rest your right hand above your right ear to add a bit more weight. Don't pull; just let the hand relax there. When you have had enough, use your right hand to push your head back to center and pause for a few breaths to allow the sensations to ebb away. Then try the other side.

Another option for increasing the stress of this lateral flexion to the cervical spine is to bring your other hand behind your back. If you want to work the left shoulder as well, try to wiggle the hand up between the shoulder blades as high as it can go. Otherwise, just let the arm rest behind you. Drop the left shoulder down as you relax the right ear over to the right shoulder. As the left shoulder drops, the sensation along the left side of the neck will intensify.

Forward Flexion

Now we work on the back side of the neck by flexing the neck forward. Most people tend to have their head hanging forward, with their ears in front of their shoulders. This is because most people spend a lot of time at a computer or watching TV: they slouch back into their chairs or couches requiring their head to come forward in order to see the screen.

Once again, come into a Shoelace pose and sit up nice and tall. Take a deep inhalation and deliberately try to lengthen the neck by pushing the crown of your head to the sky; this will create the space you need to move the head forward. Now stick your chin out and as you slowly exhale, lower your chin toward your chest. To help you sit up tall, bring your chest up to your chin with each inhale. Find that first edge, and give yourself time to open up. Again, just a couple of minutes here may be all you need at first. When you are ready to come out, use your hands to push your head back to neutral. Rest for a few breaths, relaxing the tissues you just worked.

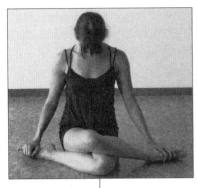

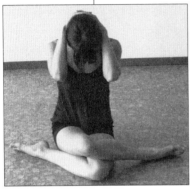

Try to find some slight variations so that you feel the stress: if you turn your head a little to the right while the chin is down, you may find the stress has moved a bit diagonally to the right side of the neck. No longer are you only feeling the back of the neck; nor are you feeling the side of the neck as we did in the lateral flexions. Now you are targeting the tissues between the side and back of the neck.

If you feel you are not at your full edge, interlace the fingers of both hands and gently rest your hands on the back of your head. Again, don't pull; the weight of your hands and arms will be enough to bring you deeper.

You may never get to a place where you feel a deep stretch here: if you have been doing yoga for a long time, you may have already stretched out those tissues enough so that what is stopping you now is compression. You have reached your ultimate limit, so there is no point pulling harder with your hands. Sometimes, compression is reached even before the chin hits the chest: the bones at the base of the skull may contact the front of the vertebrae in the neck, or two or more vertebrae may be compressing into each other. If you feel that you are stuck due to sensations in the throat area, don't force it. Just chill where you are.

One final comment about flexion of the neck: there are many poses in Yin Yoga where you are naturally flexing the neck. In Butterfly, Caterpillar, and the variations of Straddle fold, your head will be hanging down, thus the neck will be in flexion. There may be no need for you to add a specific flexion exercise for your neck, because you will be in flexion so often already. Instead, you may want to work the neck in the other directions.

Twists

We can twist our neck any time we are twisting the spine as a whole. Twisting can release tension and restore equilibrium energetically to the nervous system. Reclining Twists provide a nice chance to twist the neck, as do

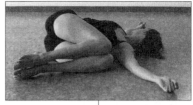

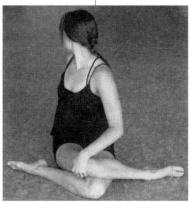

many of the seated postures. In holding twists for the neck, we are not overly working the ligaments along the spine, but more often we are affecting the fascial bags that envelop the muscles.[17]

In the Reclining Twist, as you move your legs to one side, roll your head to the other. You may find you can turn the head more if you first lift your head off the floor, turn it while it is in the air, and then lower your cheek to the floor. If you feel lightheaded at all, turn your head the other way. Or simply experiment with turning your head to both sides and then decide which way you prefer.

In Shoelace or other seated twists, the same philosophy applies. Turn the head by allowing the chin to glide over the shoulder. Find that first edge. Remember: if you are feeling it, you are doing it. No need to strain and make this a really muscular effort. Just hang out where you feel it. Time is more important than intensity. To come out, turn the head first to the other side for a moment, and then allow the rest of your body to unwind.

Backward Extension

Earlier we noted that most people tend to let their heads come forward of their shoulders and this is easily spotted in the population in general. One consequence of this head-forward position is a closing off of the front of the neck, the throat. Moving the neck backward, called extension, can help open the throat and massage the various glands located there, such as the thyroid, the four parathyroid, and the many salivary glands.

The way to extend the neck backward is quite simple, but caution is needed. There are four major arteries that bring blood to the brain: two of these are the carotid arteries, which run up the front side of the neck, and two are the vertebral arteries, which as the name implies run through the cervical vertebrae. When some people move their heads backward, their vertebrae compress the vertebral arteries and reduce the flow of blood to the brain, resulting in feelings of dizziness and light-headedness. Please note carefully the sensations you experience when you exercise your neck in any direction, but pay particular attention when you extend the neck.

Begin by sitting up nice and tall in whatever Yin Yoga pose you like, and lengthen your neck as you inhale. This will create more space to drop the head back. As you exhale, release the weight of your head. You will probably find that you stop quite quickly: this is your edge. Be content and hang out there. As discussed, some people will stop due to compression. If you have a lot of flexibility in your neck you may find that the back of your head will rest upon your upper back. Others may not hit their back but may still feel compression in the vertebrae of the neck, and you are not going to go any further. If you do not feel these points of compression, you will probably be stopped by tension in the throat. Let that just soak in for a minute or two. To come out, simply bring your head back to neutral and pause for a few breaths.

Often, when we work with the neck, we think we are curving the cervical spine, but actually all we are doing is tilting the head. For people with little neck flexibility, they disguise their lack of movement in the neck by turning, twisting or tilting their skulls on the first two cervical vertebrae. As you do any of the above movements try to feel the neck arching or twisting, rather than the head moving. The lower the vertebrae, the less range of motion it will have, so feel like you are moving your neck right from its lowest base. When you focus on the neck instead of the head, you may find that you are spreading out the intensity over more tissues: it should feel deeper. Increases in flexibility in this region will not come quickly, so be patient with the practice. Do not try to do too much too fast.

The Shoulders

The shoulder is one of the most mobile and complicated joints in the body, capable of a large variety of movements. One reason is because what we refer to as shoulder movement is really two separate movements: that of the arm and that of the scapula. The arm has six degrees of freedom,[18] while the scapula can move in eight directions.[19] If we were to analyze all the possible combinations we would have to look at forty-eight movements. We don't need to have that many postures, fortunately, to keep our shoulders in optimum condition. There are a couple of classic positions for the arms that will work the shoulders quite nicely.

Cowface Arms

From the basic Shoelace we can work the shoulders in several ways. In the classical Cowface arm position, bring your right hand high, bend the elbow, and pat yourself on the back. Bring the left hand behind your back and try to

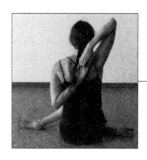 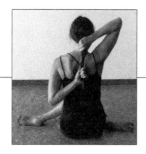 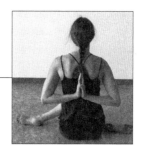

wiggle it up as high as you can. If you have the range of motion, clasp your hands; if you cannot do that, use a strap or belt and hold it with both hands. If a strap is not handy, use your ponytail. Find a place where you feel a lovely stress and let this soak in for two or three minutes. You are externally rotating, abducting and flexing the upper arm and internally rotating, adducting and extending the lower arm. The scapulae are mostly neutral.

A final variation is placing your hands in reverse prayer, also called *paschimanjali*. This is a very juicy position for both shoulders at the same time. You can do paschimanjali throughout the day: when you are walking around the house, place your arms in this position—your shoulders will loosen up quickly.

When you decide to come out of these postures, you will know right away if they worked. Your shoulders will be thanking you loudly. Come out slowly, and to release the shoulders, try pushing your hands far apart, as if you were trying to push the walls of the room apart. This is a good time to mutter "om." Now you are ready for the other side.

You may add the option of folding forward while you hold the arm position, but if you feel that folding forward reduces your stress, either in the shoulders or the hips, don't bother. If folding forward intensifies the stress nicely, then go for it. Remember, you can do this in many different basic Yin Yoga postures, such as Square Pose or Straddle.

Eagle Arms

Another variation is called Eagle Arms: bring the right elbow out in front and under the left elbow. Try to wrap the arms as tightly as you can, and see if you can bring your palms together. If you can't bring the palms together, just fake it. This is not quite Eagle Arms; eagles soar, so start to move your elbows up and away from you. Notice where you are feeling this; we are now adducting the arms but we

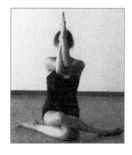

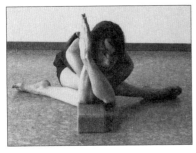

are abducting the scapulae. This pose is a lovely antidote to the tight shoulders we develop from sitting at a computer all day. As we lift the arms we are adding flexion.

If you would like to go to a deeper edge, try leaning forward and rest your elbows on a block or bolster, or hook the elbows over the front of the knees and try to get them, over time, to the floor. Keep working to slide the arms away from you. Hold for a couple of minutes. When you are finished, sit up and open the arms really wide, creating a bit of a backbend, opening the heart. Now you are ready for the other side: make sure it is the other arm that is underneath this time.

This position can be used even when you are not sitting; come onto all fours and rest your elbows on the floor, a block, or even the edge of a coffee table. Once the elbows are on something, lean away from them.

Shoulders and Arms

We have moved the arms in all 6 degrees of freedom, but we have only abducted the scapulae. This next position adducts the scapulae, providing a lovely release to the front of the chest, and puts a deep stress into the arms, especially the elbow joints. We can do this movement while still in Shoelace, but it may be deeper to try it while in Caterpillar or even in a posture we could call Sitting Swan. The Sitting Swan is an alternative way to work into the hips, if the full Swan is too much, or anytime a hip-opening pose is not accessible. Let's use Sitting Swan as the basic template for this arm variation.

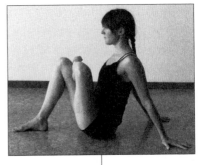

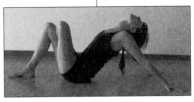

To come into the posture, take a sitting position where your legs are straight out in front of you, lean back slightly on your hands, place your left ankle over the right knee, bend the right leg and bring the heel in towards your hip. Keep the left foot flexed to support the knee. As you hold, you may find the intensity in your left hip diminishes; if so, move the hips closer to the right foot. Focus on the arms. Slowly move the hands away from you and lean into them. Notice the stress points: you may feel this entirely in the shoulders, the elbows, or the wrists. As long as you are feeling something, you are getting the benefits. Sensation is good, but don't make it sensational: when you have had enough, come out. Shake out the arms to relax them. Don't forget the other side!

A deeper option may not be available while in Sitting Swan, so try this with the legs straight out in front of you. See if you can slide the hands further behind you and bring the hands closer together. If you desire, you can drop your head back, adding extension to the neck, but remember all the neck caveats discussed earlier. Eventually, your hands will touch; this is the juiciest version. Again, don't overstay your welcome.

The Wrists

Body workers, typists, and musicians are just some of the people who suffer from repetitive stress syndrome (RSS), and often this occurs in their wrists. There is a band of fascia surrounding the wrists called the retinaculum, and there are many layers of ligaments, such as the carpal ligament, that pass over the tendons of the flexors of the fingers. Repetitive, yang-like movements of the hand can damage these yin-like tissues, creating problems with names like "carpal tunnel syndrome."[20] Yin-like exercises will help thicken and strengthen these tissues, if done properly.

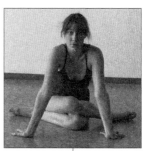

If you suffer from any form of RSS, see your health care professional before beginning treatment. As always, don't go to where it is painful, and if in any doubt, check with a professional.

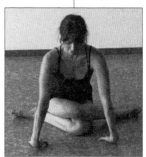

Once again we can work the hands and wrists while luxuriating in other Yin Yoga poses. Let's assume the Shoelace pose again and investigate a few options for working with the wrists in a yin-manner. Raise your hands out in front of you with the palms turned up; lower the tips of your fingers to the floor and then lean over your hands, trying to bring the heel of your palms to

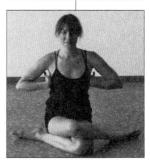

the ground. Move to the place where you feel a sensation in the inside of the forearm. If this is too much, move your hands closer toward you. If, in time, the sensations ebb away, you can move deeper by moving the hands further away from you and folding your chest toward your thighs. These sensations can be quite intense: don't stay where you feel any burning. One minute here may be enough for now. When you are done, sit back up and shake out the wrists.

Now you are ready for the other side: once again bring your hands out in front of you, but have the palms facing down. Lower your fingertips to the floor and lean forward so that you are bringing the back of your hands to the ground. You may start to feel like some sort of prehistoric, gorilla yogi with your knuckles dragging on the ground. That just means you are doing it properly. If this is too much, move your hands closer toward you: as your edge moves, try sliding the hands further away. One minute may be enough here, too. When done, sit back up and shake out the wrists.

This version of the wrist stretch is a nice counterpose for yang-yogis who love flowing vinyasas that involve lots of Up Dogs and Down Dogs. You can do these two versions of wrist stretches while in the Dragons, the Swan, in Straddle, or any seated posture.

Another variation for the back of the hands is the Seagull. Sit up tall (or come to standing if you like) and open your arms wide to the side, with the palms facing the back of the room. Now bring the back of the hands to your armpits, keeping the fingers facing the back of the room. Snuggle your hands backward a bit more. Add the juice by lowering your wings (your elbows). You may find this yin position for the wrists a nice way to end a series of sun salutations: it is similar to standing on your hands in *Padahastasana*. Hold for a minute or so, then release your hands and shake out the wrists.

These Yin Yoga positions by no means exhaust all the ways we can stress our upper body tissues. Feel free to develop other positions: remember, the principles are simple—stress the tissues, play your edges, become still, hold for time, and when finished, relax and rest the area you just worked. Also remember, we are deliberately stressing these tissues: you need to feel it. Don't be too deep—remember Goldilocks—but do be deep enough that you are getting something.

Yang Counterposes

Between yin poses many teachers suggest a bit of yang movement. This feels nice and stimulates the flow of energy in the body before the next posture. Remember, you can do too much of anything. Too much yang leads to exhaustion and depletion. Too much yin, however, leads to stagnation. Some yang between the postures helps keep stagnation from developing. Choose whatever yang movements would feel nice: let your body decide or pick something from the list below.

This list is not exhaustive, and our intention is not to describe in detail how to do yang asanas. If you wish to dive deeper into these postures or find more options, you may want to find a teacher.[21]

Cat's Breath: This is a nice counterpose to any spine work because it moves the spine in flexion and extension, getting rid of any kinks. Come onto your hands and knees and surf your breath; as you inhale, lift your head and drop your spine. As you exhale, arch your back up while you drop your chin to your chest. Begin the movement from the tailbone and allow the spine to ripple from tail to head.

Crocodile: This is a nice way to release the knees and tone the core of the body: butt and gut. It is great after Saddle pose or any hip work that stressed the knees. Basically, this is the push-up position but done on forearms. Take Sphinx pose (lying down with upper body propped up because you are on your elbows), tuck your toes under, and lift your buttocks to the same height as your shoulders. This is stage two; an easier option is stage one, where you allow your knees to stay on the ground. In either case, control your booty! Don't let your hips sag to the floor: keep the hips at the same height as your shoulders.

Down Dog and all its variations: This is probably the best counterpose after Swan or the Dragons. Down Dog stretches the back side of the body while toning the upper body. There are many ways to be a dog, but to keep it easy, come onto all fours (Cat Pose), tuck the toes under, and lift your knees off the floor. Be a happy dog: lift your tail. Push the floor away with your paws and draw your heels to the earth. They may never reach, but that is okay. Just move in that direction.

Fish: This is a fairly deep backbend and is used after intense forward folds or inversions, such as Snail Pose. Place your arms under your back as you lie down with your legs straight and together; keep the arms straight and position your hands right under the buttocks or thighs to support your lower back, elbows as close together as possible. Bend the elbows as you lift your chest. Relax the top of your head to the floor and rest on it gently. This is stage one, also known as the Minnow or Baby Fish. Stage two, if your neck is okay, is to bend your arms more and lift the chest higher until your head comes off the floor. This is a deep stretch for the throat.

Hinge: Like the Crocodile, this pose will help release the knees and tone the core of the body. It is great after Saddle pose. Lie down on your back with your hands under your buttocks or sacrum (to support the lower back.) Stage one is to keep the knees bent and drawn into the chest. On an exhalation, straighten the knees a bit and lower the feet toward the floor. As you inhale, bend the knees again and draw them back into the chest. Stage two is to do this with the legs straighter and straighter. Another variation is to alternate the legs: straighten and lower one leg at a time. Stage three is to keep the legs completely straight, and to lift them on the inhale and lower them on the exhale, all the while keeping your butt on your hands.

Tabletop (aka Hammock) or Slide: These two counterposes can be delicious any time you have been marinating in a forward fold posture, such as Butterfly or Caterpillar. With hands behind you on the floor, lift your hips up. Your feet can be on the floor with the legs bent or straight (having the legs straight turns this into Slide). Flow into this one by raising the hips and lowering them with the breath (up on inhale, down on exhale). After three or four cycles, hold the position for three or four breaths.

Windshield Wipers: This is actually a counterpose for both external rotations, such as Shoelace and for internal rotations, such as Deer, because we both internally and externally rotate the hips. Sit with your hands behind you on the floor and your feet wide apart, and drop the knees from side to side. Make sure the feet are apart! If the feet are together there is very little rotation. This can be done while lying down, too.

Feel free to spontaneously erupt into any movement that feels organic, that the body craves. But don't overdo it. Yang movements between yin postures should be brief. It is possible to create fusion classes, where we combine both yin and yang asanas in one class; however, we want to avoid constant switching from yang mode to yin mode and back again. If you are creating a fusion class, let each segment last for a while. Allow at least ten to fifteen minutes of constant yang practice or at least ten to fifteen minutes of yin practice to unfold at the same time. Do not keep switching back and forth more quickly than that. During a Yin Yoga class, keep the yang counterposes brief: thirty seconds to one minute should be enough.

NOTES

1. One of the first two Americans to learn the Ashtanga practice of Pattabhi Jois.

2. Iyengar, *Light on Yoga*, p. 129.

3. Ibid.

4. Iyengar, *Light on Yoga*, p. 150.

5. Iyengar, *Light on Yoga*, p. 88.

6. Ibid.

7. Iyengar, *Light on Yoga*, p. 170.

8. Iyengar, *Light on Yoga*, p. 93.

9. Iyengar, *Light on Yoga*, p. 239.

10. Iyengar, *Light on Yoga*, p. 125.

11. Ibid.

12. In the physiotherapy world, this is known as McKenzie therapy. For people with flexion-caused problems in the lower back (such as a slipped disk), backbends can ease the nucleus pulposus back into the middle of the disk.

13. Iyengar, *Light on Yoga*, p. 500.

14. Iyengar, *Light on Yoga*, p. 266.

15. Iyengar, *Light on Yoga*, p. 392.

16. See the section on Nadi Shodhana (p. 54) to learn how to do alternate nostril breathing.

17. We will describe these fascial bags in chapter 6, when we look at the physiology of our tissues.

18. These six movements are flexion (which means, if the arms are down at our side, moving the arms forward and up), extension (which means moving the arms back and up), abduction (moving the arms away from the side of the body), adduction (bringing the arms closer towards each other), and internal and external rotation of the arm.

19. These eight degrees of movement are adduction (the shoulder blades come together), abduction (the shoulder blades move apart), depression (where we drop the shoulder blades down the back), elevation (where we raise the shoulder blades up), upward and downward rotation, and tilting the top of the scapula backwards or forwards.

20. Carpal tunnel syndrome arises where there is pressure on the median nerve that runs under the fascia and ligaments of the wrist to the hand. There is debate whether repetitive movement actually causes carpal tunnel syndrome, and certainly there are many potential causes of this condition; the carpal tunnel may be smaller in some people, trauma or injury could have happened there, fluid retention, rheumatoid arthritis … the list goes on. However, it is well known that repetitive stress can create tendonitis, bursitis, and inflammation of the wrist joint.

21. A good option is to visit YogaJournal.com and do a search for the particular pose you are wondering about. They have a good synopsis of most of the yang asanas you are likely to come across.

chapter four Yin Yoga Flows

We have learned how to practice Yin Yoga safely and how to set an intention for our practice. We've discussed several postures and why we would want to do each one, and we have learned how to begin and end our practice. It's time now to put it all together.

The flows offered in this section are just a small sampling of what is possible, but they do provide a good representation of ways to work the main fields of the body. Feel free to experiment with them and change them around. There are ten flows here, and most of them have variations for beginners and more advanced students: choose your track deliberately. If you are a beginner, follow Track 1. Give your body, heart, and mind time to open up. The difference between Track 2 and Track 3 (which is not actually shown here) is simply the amount of time you will stay in each pose. For Track 3 simply stay in each pose longer: the whole flow could easily last a few hours! To go deeper in Yin Yoga does not mean we need newer, more difficult postures but rather, we stay longer in the simpler poses.

The ten main flows and their themes are as follows:

1. An Easy Beginner's Flow

2. A Flow for the Spine (working with the spine's 6 degrees of freedom)

3. A Flow for the Hips (working with the hips' 6 degrees of freedom)

4. A Flow for the Legs (working the four quadrants of the legs)

5. A Flow for the Shoulders, Arms, and Wrists (working the Heart and Lung lines)

6. A Flow for the Kidney and Urinary Bladder meridian lines

7. A Flow for the Liver and Gall Bladder meridian lines

8. A Flow for the Stomach and Spleen meridian lines

9. A Flow for the Whole Body (working the seldom-targeted parts of the body)

10. Wall Yin (a more restorative flow using the wall as a prop)

While there is a major theme for each flow, this does not mean that you will not work other areas of the body at the same time: you will. The theme just guides our emphasis. You may add to any of these flows your own intentions of mindfulness, breath work, healing imagery, soul work, or any other intention that you wish to invoke.

It is easy to lose track of the time as you marinate and end up doing one side longer than the other, so you may want to use a watch that can be set to beep, buzz, flash or vibrate when time is up. The total time shown for each flow is an approximation: you can decide how long you want your practice to be. The time may be a bit longer or shorter depending upon how long you wait between postures. Use a separate clock or timer to keep track of the total practice time. We have allocated about 10 percent of the practice time to Shavasana, but you may want to extend this. We have also allocated three to five minutes for the opening meditation, but again you may wish to lengthen this or even add a closing meditation after Shavasana.

1) An Easy Beginner's Flow

In this gentle, one-hour flow you'll begin by working the spine and then the hips. You will finish with twisting the spine before final relaxation. Hold each posture for three minutes, and relax the body in any way that feels comfortable for thirty to sixty seconds between asanas. You can make this into a ninety-minute practice by extending the hold times to five minutes.

AN EASY BEGINNER'S FLOW
One hour with three-minute holds

Opening Meditation

Butterfly
Counterpose: Windshield Wipers

Straddles
Fold over right leg
Fold over left leg
Fold down the middle
Counterpose: Windshield Wipers

Child's Pose (one minute)

Sphinx

Seal

Child's Pose (one minute)

Half Shoelaces
With right leg straight
With left leg straight
Counterpose: Windshield Wipers

Happy Baby

Reclining Twists
Twist to the right side
Twist to the left side

Shavasana

Finishing Meditation

2) A Flow for the Spine

This flow will move the spine through its 6 degrees of freedom: flexion, extension, lateral flexions left and right, and twists left and right. Butterfly (or Dangling) at the beginning is a mild flexion to get started. Straddle deepens the flexion over each leg and targets the sides of the spine. Caterpillar (or Snail) is the deepest flexion. We move the spine into extension via Sphinx and Seal, Bananasana provides lateral flexions, and then we finish with twists of the spine. Add movement to the neck by allowing the head to move in the same direction as the spine. For flexion, the head drops forward. For extension, the head lifts up and back. For lateral flexion, allow the ear to come toward the shoulder; and for the twists, turn the cheek to the floor. Be careful if you have neck issues. If you wish, simply extend the Track 2 hold times from Straddle onward for another two minutes.

TRACK 1 *One hour*	TRACK 2 *Ninety minutes*
Meditation for three minutes	Meditation for five minutes
Butterfly for four minutes ▷ Counterpose: Windshield Wipers	Dangling for three minutes Squat for two minutes Dangling for three minutes Squat for two minutes
Half Butterfly: fold over right leg for four minutes ▷ Counterpose: Windshield Wipers for one minute	Straddle fold over right leg for three minutes ▷ Next, add the side bend option for two minutes
Half Butterfly: fold over left leg for four minutes ▷ Counterpose: Windshield Wipers for one minute	Straddle fold over left leg for three minutes ▷ Next, add the side bend option for two minutes
	Straddle fold straight down the middle for five minutes ▷ Counterpose: Windshield Wipers for one minute
Caterpillar for four minutes ▷ Counterpose: Tabletop	Caterpillar for two minutes Snail for three minutes ▷ Counterpose: Tabletop

(Continued on the next page)

Sphinx for four minutes
  ▷ Counterpose: relax on stomach, turn head to one side, and draw that knee up beside you on the floor for one minute
	Sphinx for five minutes
	  ▷ Counterpose: relax on stomach, turn head to one side, and draw that knee up beside you on the floor for one minute

Sphinx for four more minutes
  ▷ Counterpose: relax on stomach, turn head to other side, and draw that knee up beside you on the floor for one minute
	Seal for five minutes
	  ▷ Counterpose: relax on stomach, turn head to other side, and draw that knee up beside you on the floor for one minute

Bananasana to the right for four minutes
  ▷ Counterpose: hug knees to chest and circle them
Bananasana to the left for four minutes
  ▷ Counterpose: hug knees to chest and circle the knees
	Bananasana to the right for five minutes
	Bananasana to the left for five minutes
	  ▷ Counterpose: hug knees to chest and circle them

One-knee Reclining Twist on right side for four minutes
  ▷ Counterpose: hug knees to chest and circle them
One-knee Reclining Twist on left side for four minutes
  ▷ Counterpose: hug knees to chest and circle them
	One-knee Reclining Twist on right side for five minutes
	One-knee Reclining Twist on left side for five minutes
	  ▷ Counterpose: hug knees to chest and circle them

Shavasana for seven minutes	Shavasana for ten minutes

3) A Flow for the Hips

This flow moves the hips through all 6 degrees of freedom. It includes gentle external rotation, abduction and flexion via Butterfly, abduction and flexion via Straddle, pure flexion through Caterpillar, and external rotation with Shoelace—which also combines mild adduction and flexion. With the Winged Dragon the external rotation for the front hip is combined with extension for the back hip. For Track 2 only, Camel offers a deep extension of the hip. Saddle continues some extension and adds internal rotation. Reclining Twisted Roots combines adduction with internal rotation. If you wish, simply extend the major holds in Track 2 for another two minutes. For the Dragon Cycle, choose any of the variations shown in chapter 3, or start for one minute with Baby Dragon, then move into the Dragon Flying Low for two minutes.

TRACK 1 *One hour*	TRACK 2 *Ninety minutes*
Meditation for three minutes	Meditation for five minutes
Butterfly for five minutes ▷ Counterpose: Windshield Wipers	Butterfly for five minutes ▷ Go straight into next pose
Straddle for five minutes ▷ Counterpose: Windshield Wipers	Straddle for ten minutes ▷ Counterpose: Windshield Wipers
Caterpillar for three minutes ▷ Counterpose: Tabletop	Caterpillar for three minutes ▷ Counterpose: Tabletop
Shoelace ▷ Right knee on top for three minutes ▷ Counterpose: Windshield Wipers	Shoelace ▷ Right knee on top for five minutes ▷ Counterpose: Windshield Wipers
Winged Dragon ▷ Step right foot forward and hold for two minutes ▷ Counterpose: step back to Down Dog	Dragon Cycle for five minutes ending in Winged Dragon ▷ Step right foot forward ▷ Hold Winged Dragon for two minutes ▷ Counterpose: step back to Down Dog
Shoelace ▷ Left knee on top for three minutes ▷ Counterpose: Windshield Wipers	Shoelace ▷ Left knee on top for five minutes ▷ Counterpose: Windshield Wipers
Winged Dragon ▷ Step left foot forward and hold for two minutes ▷ Counterpose: step back to Down Dog	Dragon Cycle for five minutes ending in Winged Dragon ▷ Step left foot forward ▷ Hold Winged Dragon for two minutes ▷ Counterpose: step back to Down Dog
	Camel ▷ Counterpose: Child's Pose ▷ Do Camel twice, holding each one for two minutes ▷ Keep the first Camel easy
Half Saddle ▷ Sit on bolster with right leg forward for three minutes ▷ Switch to left leg forward for three minutes ▷ Counterpose: Child's Pose for one minute	Saddle, sitting between feet, for five minutes ▷ Counterpose: Crocodile for one minute

(Continued on the next page)

Reclining Twist (Twisted Roots) ▷ Twist to the right side for three minutes ▷ Twist to the left side for three minutes ▷ Counterpose: hug knees in and circle them	Reclining Twist (Twisted Roots) ▷ Twist to the right side for five minutes ▷ Twist to the left side for five minutes Counterpose: hug knees in and circle them
Shavasana for seven minutes	Shavasana for ten minutes

4) A Flow for the Legs

The upper legs have four sides: the top (quadriceps), inner legs (adductors), backs of legs (hamstrings), and outside (IT band and abductors.) This flow targets the fascial bags within each of the major muscle groups in all four quadrants. By targeting the fascia through long-held stresses, we can help lengthen the whole myofascial group and improve our range of motion and health of these tissues. The key to this flow is to relax: keep the muscles soft and work with your ocean breath. Again, if you wish, simply luxuriate in each position for a couple more minutes.

TRACK 1 *One hour*	TRACK 2 *Ninety minutes*
Meditation for three minutes	Meditation for five minutes
Butterfly for three minutes	Butterfly for five minutes
Straddle for seven minutes	Straddle for ten minutes
Caterpillar for three minutes	Caterpillar for five minutes
Swan ▷ Full Swan with right knee forward for two minutes ▷ Sleeping Swan for two minutes	Swan ▷ Full Swan with right knee forward for two minutes ▷ Sleeping Swan for three minutes
Shoelace with left knee on top for three minutes ▷ Counterpose: Windshield Wipers	Shoelace with left knee on top for five minutes ▷ Counterpose: Windshield Wipers
Swan ▷ Full Swan with left knee forward for two minutes ▷ Sleeping Swan for two minutes	Swan ▷ Full Swan with left knee forward for two minutes ▷ Sleeping Swan for three minutes
Shoelace with right knee on top for three minutes ▷ Counterpose: Windshield Wipers	Shoelace with right knee on top for five minutes ▷ Counterpose: Windshield Wipers

(Continued on the next page)

Saddle, sitting between feet, for three minutes ▷ If Saddle is not available, do Baby Dragon on each side for two minutes ▷ Counterpose: Hinge	Saddle, sitting between feet, for five minutes ▷ If Saddle is not available, do Baby Dragon on each side for four minutes ▷ Counterpose: Hinge
Bananasana to the right for three minutes ▷ Counterpose: hug knees to chest and circle them Bananasana to the left for three minutes ▷ Counterpose: hug knees to chest and circle them	Bananasana to the right for four minutes ▷ Counterpose: hug knees to chest and circle them Bananasana to the left for four minutes ▷ Counterpose: hug knees to chest and circle them
One-knee Reclining Twist on right side for one minute ▷ Counterpose: hug knees to chest and circle them One-knee Reclining Twist on left side for one minute ▷ Counterpose: hug knees to chest and circle them	One-knee Reclining Twist on right side with the top leg (left) extended out to the side for three minutes ▷ Counterpose: hug knees to chest and circle them One-knee Reclining Twist on left side with the top leg (right) extended out to the side for three minutes ▷ Counterpose: hug knees to chest and circle them
Shavasana for seven minutes	Shavasana for ten minutes

5) A Flow for the Shoulders, Arms, and Wrists

This flow works the spine and hips at the same time that it works the shoulders via Eagle Arms and Cowface Arms, the elbows via Sitting Swan, and the wrists via Butterfly or Straddle. While we stress these upper body tissues, we will also stimulate the upper body meridian lines, especially the Heart and Lungs. Review the asanas we will be using for the shoulders, arms, and wrists (see Chapter 3) to help you choose the options that work best. Remember, if you feel any tingling in the fingers, back off or come out of the pose.

TRACK 1 *One hour*	TRACK 2 *Ninety minutes*
Meditation for three minutes	Meditation for five minutes
Child's Pose with arms overhead for three minutes	Frog ▷ Start in Tadpole for two minutes ▷ Move hips forward to full Frog for three minutes
Anahatasana for three minutes	Anahatasana for four minutes
Sphinx for three minutes ▷ Counterpose: relax on stomach, turn head to one side, and draw that knee up beside you on the floor for one minute	Sphinx for five minutes ▷ Counterpose: relax on stomach, turn head to one side, and draw that knee up beside you on the floor for one minute
Seal for two minutes ▷ Counterpose: relax on stomach, turn head to other side, and draw that knee up beside you on the floor for one minute	Seal pose for five minutes ▷ Counterpose: relax on stomach, turn head to other side and draw that knee up beside you on the floor for one minute
Half Shoelace with right leg on top, left leg extended ▷ Cowface Arms with right hand behind back for two minutes ▷ Counterpose: Release arms and push hands apart ▷ Eagle Arms with left arm under the right for two minutes ▷ Counterpose: Release arms and push hands apart	Shoelace with right leg on top ▷ Cowface Arms with right hand behind back for three minutes ▷ Counterpose: Release arms and push hands apart ▷ Eagle Arms with left arm under the right for two minutes ▷ Counterpose: Release arms and push hands apart
Stretch legs out straight and lean back on the hands for one minute ▷ Or do Sitting Swan variation	Sitting Swan with right ankle on left knee ▷ Leaning on hands, move the hands as far away as they can go ▷ Hold for two minutes
Half Shoelace with left leg on top, right leg extended ▷ Cowface Arms with left hand behind back for two minutes ▷ Counterpose: Release arms and push hands apart ▷ Eagle Arms with right arm under the left for two minutes ▷ Counterpose: Release arms and push hands apart	Shoelace with left leg on top ▷ Cowface Arms with left hand behind back for three minutes ▷ Counterpose: Release arms and push hands apart ▷ Eagle Arms with right arm under the left for two minutes ▷ Counterpose: Release arms and push hands apart

(Continued on the next page)

Stretch legs out straight and lean back on the hands for one minute ▷ Or do Sitting Swan variation	Sitting Swan with left ankle on right knee ▷ Leaning on hands, move the hands as far away as they can go (see if you can bring them together) ▷ Hold for two minutes
Butterfly ▷ Bring hands out in front, turn palms up, and lower fingers to the floor. Lean forward until the heel of the palm is near the floor or until you feel stress in the inner forearm. Hold for one minute. ▷ Release and shake out the wrists. ▷ Bring hands out in front, turn palms down, and lower fingers to the floor. Lean forward until the back of the wrist is near the floor or until you feel stress in the back of the wrist. Hold for one minute. ▷ Release and shake out the wrists ▷ Stay in Butterfly for another three minutes.	Straddle ▷ Bring hands out in front, turn palms up, and lower fingers to the floor. Lean forward until the heel of the palm is near the floor or until you feel stress in the inner forearm. Hold for two minutes. ▷ Release and shake out the wrists. ▷ Bring hands out in front, turn palms down, and lower fingers to the floor. Lean forward until the back of the wrist is near the floor or until you feel stress in the back of the wrist. Hold for two minutes. ▷ Release and shake out the wrists ▷ Stay in Straddle for another five minutes.
One-knee Reclining Twist on right side for two minutes with left arm alongside ear ▷ Counterpose: hug knees to chest and circle them One-knee Reclining Twist on left side for two minutes with right arm alongside ear ▷ Counterpose: hug knees to chest and circle them	One-knee Reclining Twist on right side for five minutes with left arm alongside ear ▷ Counterpose: hug knees to chest and circle them One-knee Reclining Twist on left side for five minutes with right arm alongside ear ▷ Counterpose: hug knees to chest and circle them
Shavasana for seven minutes	Shavasana for ten minutes

6) A Flow for the Kidney and Urinary Bladder Meridian Lines

This flow includes forward and backbends that work these lines very well. The Track 2 flow adds more stimulation to the inner groins. Any flow focusing on the spine will be very effective at stimulating and nourishing the kidneys. Note that we start with extension of the spine; this allows a nice compression of the kidneys. The Kidneys are the home of Jing,[1] which is stored in the Kidneys and from there is sent out to all the other organs. We can enhance the flow of energy along these lines with our breath and attention, as described in chapter 2.

TRACK 1 *One hour*	TRACK 2 *Ninety minutes*
Meditation for three minutes	Meditation for five minutes
Sphinx for five minutes ▷ Counterpose: relax on stomach, turn head to one side, and draw that knee up beside you on the floor for one minute	Sphinx for five minutes ▷ Counterpose: relax on stomach, turn head to one side, and draw that knee up beside you on the floor for one minute
Saddle, sitting on feet or a block, for three minutes ▷ If Saddle is not available, do Half Saddle on each side for two minutes ▷ If Saddle still doesn't work, do another round of Sphinx ▷ Counterpose: Child's Pose	Saddle, sitting on feet or a block, for six minutes ▷ If Saddle is not available, do Half Saddle on each side for three minutes ▷ Counterpose: Crocodile for one minute
Sphinx, or Seal if doable, for five minutes ▷ Counterpose: relax on stomach, turn head to one side, and draw that knee up beside you on the floor for one minute	Seal pose for five minutes ▷ Counterpose: relax on stomach, turn head to one side, and draw that knee up beside you on the floor for one minute
Butterfly for four minutes	Butterfly for five minutes
Half Butterfly: fold over right leg for three minutes ▷ Counterpose: Windshield Wipers for one minute Half Butterfly: fold over left leg for three minutes ▷ Counterpose: Windshield Wipers for one minute Straddle fold straight down the middle for three minutes ▷ Counterpose: Windshield Wipers for one minute	Straddle fold over right leg for five minutes Straddle fold over left leg for five minutes Straddle fold straight down the middle for five minutes ▷ Counterpose: Windshield Wipers for one minute
Caterpillar for five minutes ▷ Counterpose: Tabletop	Caterpillar for two minutes Snail for three minutes ▷ Counterpose: Tabletop
	Anahatasana for four minutes

(Continued on the next page)

	Dragon Cycle: start with right foot forward
	▷ Baby Dragon for one minute
	▷ High Flying Dragon for two minutes
	▷ Winged Dragon for two minutes
	▷ Dragon Splits for one minute
	▷ Counterpose: Down Dog for one minute
	▷ Do the other side with left foot forward
Reclining Twist (Twisted Roots) ▷ Twist to the right side for four minutes ▷ Twist to the left side for four minutes ▷ Counterpose: hug knees in and circle them	Reclining Twist (Twisted Roots) ▷ Twist to the right side for five minutes ▷ Twist to the left side for five minutes Counterpose: hug knees in and circle them
Shavasana for seven minutes	Shavasana for ten minutes

7) A Flow for the Liver and Gall Bladder Meridian Lines

Any flows that include hip openers and twists stimulate the Liver and Gall Bladder lines very well. We can enhance the flow of energy along these lines with our breath and our attention, as described in chapter 7.

To help activate the Liver and Gallbladder it is useful to activate the Kidneys, too. The Kidneys' Jing energy supports all the internal organs. You will notice that we stimulate the Kidneys early in this flow via the first Sphinx and Seal poses.

TRACK 1 *One hour*	TRACK 2 *Ninety minutes*
Meditation for three minutes	Meditation for five minutes
	Frog: Begin in Tadpole for two minutes Move into full Frog for three minutes ▷ Counterpose: slide onto your stomach for one minute
Sphinx, or Seal if doable, for five minutes ▷ Counterpose: relax on stomach, turn head to one side, and draw that knee up beside you on the floor for one minute	Sphinx for five minutes ▷ Counterpose: relax on stomach, turn head to one side, and draw that knee up beside you on the floor for one minute
	Seal for five minutes ▷ Counterpose: relax on stomach, turn head to one side, and draw that knee up beside you on the floor for one minute
Swan ▷ Full Swan with right knee forward for one minute ▷ Sleeping Swan for three minutes ▷ Child's Pose for one minute	Swan ▷ Full Swan with right knee forward for two minutes ▷ Sleeping Swan for three minutes ▷ Lean to your right and come into Shoelace
Shoelace with left knee on top for five minutes ▷ For first half of the time, twist to the left ▷ For last half of the time, side bend to the right ▷ Windshield Wipers for one minute	Shoelace with left knee on top for five minutes ▷ For first half of the time, twist to the left ▷ For last half of the time, side bend to the left ▷ Windshield Wipers for one minute
Swan ▷ Full Swan with left knee forward for one minute ▷ Sleeping Swan for three minutes ▷ Child's Pose for one minute	Swan ▷ Full Swan with left knee forward for two minutes ▷ Sleeping Swan for three minutes ▷ Lean to your left and come into Shoelace
Shoelace with right knee on top for five minutes ▷ For first half of the time, twist to the right ▷ For last half of the time, side bend to the left ▷ Windshield Wipers for one minute	Shoelace with right knee on top for five minutes ▷ For first half of the time, twist to the right ▷ For last half of the time, side bend to the right ▷ Windshield Wipers for one minute

(Continued on the next page)

Straddle fold over right leg for three minutes ▷ Windshield Wipers Straddle fold over left leg for three minutes ▷ Windshield Wipers Straddle fold straight down the middle for three minutes ▷ Windshield Wipers for one minute	Straddle fold over right leg for three minutes ▷ Next, add the side bend option for two more minutes Straddle fold over left leg for three minutes ▷ Next, add the sidebend option for two more minutes Straddle fold straight down the middle for five minutes ▷ Windshield Wipers for one minute
Bananasana to the right for three minutes ▷ Counterpose: hug knees to chest and circle them Bananasana to the left for three minutes ▷ Counterpose: hug knees to chest and circle them	Bananasana to the right for five minutes ▷ Counterpose: hug knees to chest and circle them Bananasana to the left for five minutes ▷ Counterpose: hug knees to chest and circle them
One-knee Reclining Twist on right side for two minutes ▷ Counterpose: hug knees to chest and circle them One-knee Reclining Twist on left side for two minutes ▷ Counterpose: hug knees to chest and circle them	One-knee Reclining Twist on right side with the top leg (left) extended out to the side for two minutes ▷ Bend top leg and come into one-knee twist for three minutes ▷ Counterpose: hug knees to chest and circle them One-knee Reclining Twist on left side with the top leg (right) extended out to the side for two minutes ▷ Bend top leg and come into one-knee twist for three minutes ▷ Counterpose: hug knees to chest and circle them
Shavasana for seven minutes	Shavasana for ten minutes

8) A Flow for the Stomach and Spleen Meridian Lines

Any flows that include spinal or hip extensions can nourish the Stomach and Spleen. Deep twisting of the spine can also help to massage the internal organs. We can enhance the flow of energy along these lines with our breath and our attention, as described in chapter 7.

To help activate the Spleen and Stomach it is useful to activate the Kidneys, too. The Kidneys' Jing energy supports all the internal organs. You will notice that we stimulate the Kidneys early in this flow via the first Sphinx and Seal poses, but we start with Child's Pose to compress the belly.

TRACK 1 *One hour*	TRACK 2 *Ninety minutes*
Meditation for three minutes	Meditation for five minutes
Child's Pose for three minutes	Child's Pose for five minutes
Sphinx, building up to Seal if doable, for five minutes ▷ Counterpose: relax on stomach, turn head to one side, and draw that knee up beside you on the floor for one minute	Sphinx for five minutes ▷ Counterpose: relax on stomach, turn head to one side, and draw that knee up beside you on the floor for one minute
Saddle, sitting between feet or on a block, for four minutes ▷ If Saddle is not available, do Half Saddle on each side for two minutes ▷ If Saddle still doesn't work, do another round of Sphinx ▷ Counterpose: Child's Pose	Saddle, sitting between feet, for six minutes ▷ If Saddle is not available, do Half Saddle on each side for three minutes ▷ Counterpose: Crocodile for one minute
	Seal for five minutes ▷ Counterpose: relax on stomach, turn head to one side, and draw that knee up beside you on the floor for one minute
Shoelace with left knee on top ▷ Twist to the left for two minutes ▷ Fold forward for two minutes ▷ Windshield Wipers ▷ Other side: right knee on top, twist to the right for two minutes, then fold forward for two minutes	Shoelace with left knee on top ▷ Twist to the left for two minutes ▷ Fold forward for three minutes ▷ Windshield Wipers ▷ Other side: right knee on top, twist to the right for two minutes, then fold forward for three minutes
	Straddle Fold down the middle for ten minutes
Caterpillar for three minutes	Caterpillar for five minutes
Dragon Cycle: start with right foot forward ▷ Baby Dragon for one minute ▷ Low Flying Dragon for one minute ▷ Dragon Splits for one minute ▷ Child's Pose for one minute ▷ Do the other side with left foot forward	Dragon Cycle: start with right foot forward ▷ Baby Dragon for one minute ▷ High Flying Dragon for two minutes ▷ Low Flying Dragon for two minutes ▷ Dragon Splits for one minute ▷ Counterpose: Down Dog for one minute ▷ Do the other side with left foot forward

(Continued on the next page)

One-knee Reclining Twist on right side for four minutes ▷ Counterpose: hug knees to chest and circle them One-knee Reclining Twist on left side for four minutes ▷ Counterpose: hug knees to chest and circle them	One-knee Reclining Twist on right side for four minutes One-knee Reclining Twist on left side for four minutes ▷ Counterpose: hug knees to chest and circle them
Shavasana for seven minutes	Shavasana for ten minutes

9) A Flow for the Whole Body

This flow targets many areas of the body that get missed in our normal yoga practices, yin or yang. We will work from the tips of the toes to the top of the head and touch many places in between. Try it all: don't skip the face yoga practice.[2] Heart tapping, which we do at the beginning, stimulates the immune system. The thymus gland is located right above the heart and beneath the sternum: when we tap, we stimulate the cells in the thymus, which matures the white blood stem cells. You can also imagine that you are massaging your heart. Zipper requires you to bring the soles of your feet together and interlace your toes, thus stimulating all six lower body meridians, which begin or end in the toes.[3] If you are not familiar with poses like Ankle Stretch, Toe Squat, and Happy Baby, review them in chapter 3. The poses or movements not found there are described in the flow's narrative. We end with a lovely yang movement called Tantrumasana. For Track 1, hold for the minimum times shown; for Track 2, hold for the longer periods.

A WHOLE BODY YIN WORKOUT
Sixty to seventy-five minutes

Meditation for three minutes

Heart Tapping for two minutes
- ▷ Use the tips of the fingers of your right hand to tap along your sternum. Go slowly at first.

Butterfly with toes in Zipper for five minutes
- ▷ Neck circles: Allow your head to drop to the right shoulder, then lower your chin to your chest and raise your left ear to the left shoulder. Repeat these half circles several times.
- ▷ Try making a full circle by dropping your head back. Allow your chin to make a full circle. Switch directions after two or three orbits.
- ▷ Shoulder Circles: keeping your head centered, draw your shoulders forward, up, back, and down. Let your arms move freely. Switch directions after two or three orbits.

Dangling for three minutes
- ▷ Track 1: If Dangling is too intense, do Caterpillar instead.

Squat for three minutes
- ▷ Track 1: If Squat is too intense, do a tight Butterfly, where the feet are drawn in close to the body.

Toe Squat for five minutes
- ▷ During this pose, we have time to work the shoulders and our face. First, bring your arms into Cowface, with the left hand behind you, and the right arm up in the air. If you can't clasp, use a strap or a belt. Hold for two minutes.
- ▷ For the face yoga, allow the biggest, goofiest smile you can manage to envelop your face.
- ▷ Release the arms and move into Eagle Arms with the right arm underneath. Move the elbows up and away. Hold for two minutes.
- ▷ While in Eagle Arms, the next face posture is the Scream: open your eyes and mouth as wide as you can. Stretch!
- ▷ Release the arms straight up in the air, interlace the fingers, and push the palms away for one minute. Stick your tongue out so that it touches your chin, look up, and roar like a lion.
- ▷ When done, give your scalp a nice massage for one minute.

Ankle Stretch for two minutes
- ▷ Counterpose: Step back to Crocodile for one minute.

(Continued on the next page)

Toe Squat: part two, for five minutes
  ▷ Bring your arms into Cowface, with the right hand behind you and the left arm up in the air. If you can't clasp, use a strap or belt. Hold for two minutes.
  ▷ For the face yoga, keep your head centered and slide your face to the right as far as you can. Look to the right, but don't turn your head. Move your jaw to the right. You will feel like Popeye.[4]
  ▷ Release the arms and move into Eagle Arms with the left arm underneath. Move the elbows up and away. Hold for two minutes.
  ▷ While in Eagle Arms, keep your head centered and slide your face to the left as far as you can.
  ▷ Release the arms straight up in the air, interlace the fingers, and push the palms away for one minute. Stick your tongue out so that it touches your chin, look up, and roar like a lion.
  ▷ When done, give your scalp a nice massage for one minute.

Ankle Stretch for two minutes
  ▷ Counterpose: Crocodile for one minute

Sphinx, building up to Seal if doable, for five minutes
  ▷ Counterpose: Child's Pose for one minute

Happy Baby for three to five minutes

Bananasana to the right for three to five minutes
  ▷ Counterpose: hug knees to chest and circle them

Bananasana to the left for three to five minutes
  ▷ Counterpose: hug knees to chest and circle them

Reclining Twist (Twisted Roots)
  ▷ Twist to the right side for four minutes
  ▷ Twist to the left side for four minutes
  ▷ Counterpose: hug knees in and circle them

Tantrumasana
  ▷ Lying on your back, bend your knees so that your feet are flat on the floor. Place hands beside your feet, palms flat on the floor.
  ▷ For thirty seconds, slap the floor with your hands and feet as fast as you can.
  ▷ Pause for fifteen seconds and then repeat for twenty seconds.
  ▷ Pause again for fifteen seconds and do a final burst for ten seconds.
  ▷ Feel free to chant as you make as much noise as you can. Go fast! Channel your inner brat.

Shavasana for seven minutes

10) Wall Yin

Ever have one of those days where you didn't want to do anything but collapse? Your get-up-and-go has got up and went? Your yoga buddy, whom you rely on for moral support, has bailed on you? Where can you go for that support now? Well, it may be as close as that wall over there! Put on some soothing music, clear a space by your longest wall, grab a watch (preferably with a timer) and a cushion or two, and settle into some wall yin.

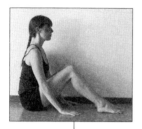

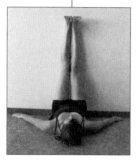

Wall Butterfly: Like all yoga journeys, you can start with a brief meditation, but this time with the wall supporting your feet. The easiest way to get into this position may be to sit sideways against the wall and then swivel: swing your legs up the wall and lie down. Next, try to snuggle your buttocks to the corner of the wall and the floor. Bring your feet together and let your heels come as low as they can, and allow the knees to go as wide as they can. Since this is your meditation position, place your hands where you feel most comfortable: either over your heart or your belly (or one hand over each), or let your arms fall to the sides. Wait here for as long as your intuition suggests. Breath, allow a few sighs to slip out, and be present.

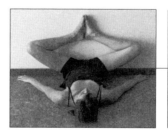
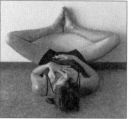

Wall Caterpillar: From Wall Butterfly, simply straighten your legs up the wall. If you find that you can't keep your legs straight, wiggle a little away from the wall. A nice option here may be to place a cushion under your sacrum. Hold this position between three and ten minutes. It is very restorative and great for people who have been on their feet all day.

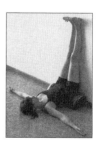

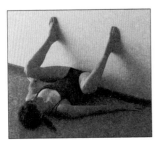

Wall Squat (aka Wall Happy Baby): Starting from the legs straight up the wall, bend both knees and slide your feet down. Have the feet comfortably apart, which for you may be approximately hip width. If the feet and knees are wider than hip-width apart, the pose gets juicier. Now your buttocks may have lifted off the floor when you slid your feet down: for some people this is quite all right and they like the hips up a bit. Others may not like this because it puts too much stress into the sacrum. Feel free to slide a bit away from the wall so that your sacrum can be flat on the floor. The intention here is to wake up the hip sockets, so as long as you are feeling something there, you are getting the pose. Three to five minutes here should be enough. For the last minute or so, try coming into the traditional Happy Baby by grabbing your feet or holding the backs of your thighs and pulling your knees to the floor. When you have had enough, straighten the legs up against the wall and release any tension from the previous posture. Wiggle, move, and do whatever feels organic. Try a version of Tantrumasana that you may have perfected when you were a child. Let your arms and legs flail in the air!

Wall Straddle: You will need a bit of space for this one, especially if you are quite flexible. Start with your legs straight up the wall (or your variation of that) and then let gravity draw the legs apart, your feet sliding 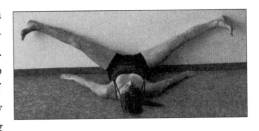 down the wall. Reach the Goldilocks' position where the sensations are just right. When you want a little more, try resting your hands on your inner thighs. No need to pull: let your muscles relax. Stay here for three to five minutes. When you are ready to come out, use your hands to push your legs together, like closing a book. Wiggle and move. Remember, a bit of yang movement between the yin poses helps to free up stuck energy.

Wall Eye (of the needle): We will start on the right side; however, if your left hip is the more open one, feel free to start on the left side first. Begin with your legs straight up the wall and then place your right ankle on your left knee. Since you are upside-down, the words above and below can be confusing,

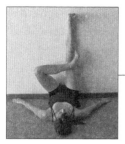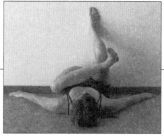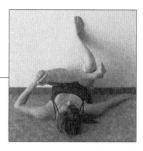

but ideally we want the ankle just below the knee, which means closer to the floor or on your thigh, but not your shin. Flex the right foot, which helps to support the knee, and then slowly bend the straight leg, sliding the foot down the wall. See if you can get to a position in which your left foot is at the same height as the left knee. This is the position of maximum stress for the hip.

If you need to, slide your buttocks away from the wall so that the sacrum can remain flat on the floor. Either way can be okay: you may want to stay there and let your hips be off the floor, or you may choose to move a bit away from the wall until your sacrum is again flat on the floor. One position is not better than the other. Notice the differences in where you feel each variation, and then choose which one you want to do.

Ease into this in stages: don't slide your left foot down the wall too quickly. You can also use your right hand to press into your knee and wing it out a few times to loosen up the joint before you hold in stillness. Hold here for three to five minutes, and come out of the pose by moving into a twist.[5]

Reclining Twist: From the eye of the needle we come into a reclining twist by simply lowering the legs and hips to the left, to the floor, while keeping the upper body where it is. You may want to spread your arms wide apart to help anchor your shoulders, then drop your right foot and left knee to the left and find a comfortable twist. Keeping your left foot (ideally the top of it) against the wall

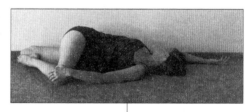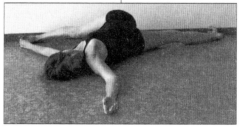

will keep your knees closer to your chest, which can make this a deeper twist.

Even more challenging is to straighten both legs in opposite directions and have the feet still pressing against the wall (as shown in the previous picture). Hold here for three to five minutes. Come out of this pose by returning the legs up the wall and shaking them out for a bit.

Wall Eye (left side): Do the previous two postures again but on the other side this time. Start with your left ankle on your right knee. When done, go into the twist.

Reclining Twist (right side): Drop both your left foot and right knee to the right side.

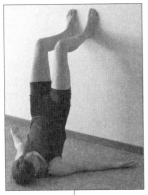

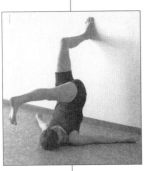

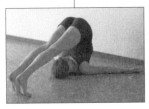

Wall Arch: Skip this posture if you don't want to invert today. The standard cautions and contra-indications for inversions apply: folks with neck issues, high blood pressure, glaucoma, diabetes, women who are menstruating, or anyone who just doesn't want to go upside down, leave this one out! If you are ready to try it, return your legs straight up the wall.

Slide both feet down the wall, as if you were coming into Wall Squat, but don't lower the feet too far: 12–18 inches should be enough. Place your hands beside you, palms pressing into the floor. Press both feet into the wall and lift your hips high off the floor. Come into an arch. Keep your hands on the floor. Don't worry if your hips are not over your shoulders. By pressing into the wall with your legs instead of using your back muscles or arms you should find it easy to stay upside-down for quite a while. Stay here for a minute before trying the second variation.

The second variation is to allow your right foot to come off the wall and let that leg dangle over your head toward the floor. Keep the left foot on the wall. Stay here only if your neck is not complaining. After a minute or so, switch legs.

The final variation, again not for everyone, is to have both legs fall over your head and come into Snail pose for the last minute or two. Come out of Snail by returning one leg at a time to the arch, and then lower down slowly. You may want to shake out your legs or do a mild spinal lift here to relax your spine.

Wall Sphinx: We finish in Sphinx but with our shins up against the wall. To come into this, roll over onto your belly. Bend your knees and scoot yourself back to the wall so that your knees are now at the corner between the wall and the floor. Your shins will be against the wall. Clasp your elbows with the opposite hands. For a few minutes allow the back to soak into this shape, and if you want a bit more compression or sensation in the lumbar spine, feel free to rest your elbows on a cushion. Stay for three to five minutes. The deepest version of this pose is to extend the arms into Wall Seal.

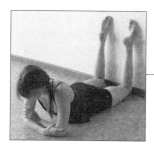 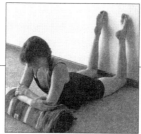 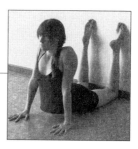

Shavasana and Closing Meditation: Now relax! Since this whole sequence has been rather relaxing already, you may choose to skip a reclining Shavasana and just sit quietly for several minutes.

NOTES

1. Jing is the generative energy, according to Daoist philosophy. It is described in detail in chapter 7.

2. There are more than forty muscles in our face, depending on how you count them. We can do yoga for these muscles just as we can for any others. Who says our hamstrings are more important that our zygomaticus minor?

3. If you can't interlace your toes, that is not a good sign! You are probably wearing unsensible shoes. There is an old Daoist saying, "Man with open toes has open mind." This applies to women too! If you can't interlace your toes, use your fingers or balls of cotton as spreaders. This will feel really nice when you come out of the pose.

4. Popeye, for those who do not know him, is a famous American Zen master, but unfortunately a fictional one. He often would say, "I am what I am." Brilliant.

5. A note from Lorien in the YinYoga.com Forum on this pose: "The students with really open hips may need a little help to get any sensation in Eye-of-the-needle pose. Let's say the right foot is resting on the left thigh; as I bend my left knee and slide my foot down the wall, my right knee falls into my chest and I feel no sensation around my hips unless I open my right knee toward the wall. I've found that if I brace my right elbow on the floor and prop open my right thigh with my hand, I can hold this position without a lot of muscular effort. Some students place a block on their ribcage to prop the thigh, but I don't like what that does to my breath. Did I mention yet how much I love using the wall?"

chapter five Special Situations

Yin Yoga is softer, yielding, and nourishing—many of the qualities that draw people to restorative yoga. While restorative yoga incorporates many yin elements, the form of Yin Yoga described in this book is not restorative yoga: the intentions are quite different. Restorative yoga principally tries to heal specific problems and regain health, while Yin Yoga makes an assumption that you are already healthy and want to go beyond this to wellness and optimal health. We can, however, use the system of Yin Yoga described here to help us out when we are not in optimal shape or when we have special conditions to take into consideration.

There are numerous special conditions that arise in the population of yoga students. In the Forum at YinYoga.com students often ask questions about how Yin Yoga may help with their own special injury or circumstance, and through community feedback valuable suggestions are made. In this chapter we will go over three of the most common issues: knees and hips, the lower back, and pregnancy and fertility. What is presented is far from the final word, but it will give some guidance. Feel free to ask about your own situation in the forum or offer wisdom for those who are working through their own challenges. Remember, talk to your health care provider before trying any of these suggestions!

Yin Yoga predominantly targets the area from the knees to the navel. Often, knee issues are caused by hip problems; working to safely open the hips can reduce knee pain. Let's start from the ground and work our way up, starting first with the knees.

Hip & Knee Issues

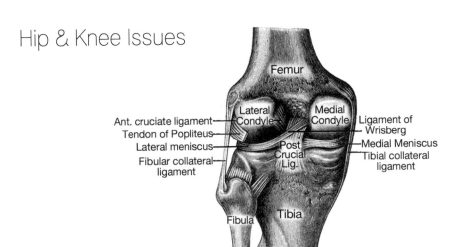

The most common problems with the knees are tears to the ligaments and cartilage, and arthritis. Although we cannot cover all the pathologies related to the knees, we will discuss one particular problem that crops up often in yoga classes: torn menisci.

The knee is a complex joint with many ligaments wrapping it to give it structural support. Between the two bones that form the knee joint (the femur and tibia) there are two C-shaped cushions of cartilage called the menisci. These allow the two bones to join together snugly and provide some cushioning support so that the ends of the bones do not come into abrasive contact.

When we externally rotate our leg with the knee bent, pressure can build up in the inner knee. If the hips are tight and won't easily rotate (common for most Westerners), the stress from the external rotation tends to go to the next joint, which is the knee. Fortunately, our bodies are designed to warn us with pain when the stress in the knee joint becomes dangerous. Unfortunately, we don't always listen, we push into the pain, and the result is a torn meniscus.

If the pain is severe and continuous, surgery may be the only choice. If the pain is minor and manageable, you can live with the tear, but what else can you do to make sure you don't make it worse? Yin Yoga! By working to open the hips, slowly and over time, we can reduce stress on the menisci and minimize discomfort.

We can use Yin Yoga to open the hips and reduce knee stress in two ways: by doing lots of the hip-opening postures during our asana practice and by living on the floor. Poses that are great for opening the hips include Shoelace, Square, Swan, and the Dragons. Remember, we want zero tolerance of any pain in the knees with these poses. Living on the floor is the other way to open the knees. A major cause of tight hips is the fact that we spend so much time sitting in chairs. Sit on the floor as often as possible. Don't worry about how to do it; change your posture as frequently as you like—just get down there. Sit cross-legged sometimes, stretch one leg out for a while, have both legs out, come into Shoelace, wiggle back into Swan: it doesn't matter.

Hip openers avoid stressing the knees further; however, sometimes stressing the knees is exactly what we do need. Stress can stimulate healing, if done intelligently. Again, check with your doctor and listen to your body. Straddle is one example: when the legs are spread wide apart, there is a lovely tugging on the medial collateral ligament, which runs along the inside of the knee. The medial meniscus is part of that ligament, so when you feel a nice stress there, you are helping to stimulate whatever fibroblasts and chondrocytes are around. Chondrocytes are the cells the build new cartilage; fibroblasts build new ligaments. Again, if there is pain when you do this, stop and bring the legs closer together.

A highly recommended pose for knee issues is Saddle, but you do not have to recline for this version. In the yang yoga world, this is known as the Thunderbolt or *Vajrasana*; this is also known as a variation of Hero Pose or *Virasana*. Basically, this is just sitting on your heels.[1] If it is not possible, put a couple of blocks between your feet and sit on them. If your ankles complain, try putting a folded towel under them. This pose will stress the knees and can be very therapeutic for the knee caps, ankles, and arch of the foot. We can make it juicier, if that is appropriate: try rolling up a cloth or towel and tucking it tightly behind the knees; this will, over time, create more space in the knee joint. Many people with meniscus problems have found this variation highly beneficial.

One of the biggest concerns for the knees is osteoarthritis, which is painful and very damaging to the joint. The condition has many causes but one is a yang-like rubbing of the bones and cartilage with little or no lubricant between them, causing the cartilage to wear away. One way to help rebuild the bones is to stress them. This is discussed in more detail in the next chapter. We have to be careful now: too much stress makes the condition worse, but no stress also makes the condition worse. As always, check in with your health care provider and let her know what you are planning to do.

Hip Replacement

The most common problems with our hips are tears to the ligaments and the labrum, and osteoporosis.[2] We will discuss how Yin Yoga can help with

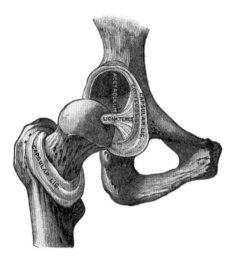

osteoporosis in the next chapter. Now, let's look at how to help strengthen and lengthen the ligaments of the hips.

Often students will complain about how tight their hips are, and it is no wonder—in the West our hips are tight! The joint has shrink wrapped to a very small range of motion, especially in rotation. The joint capsule, made up of connective tissue, and the ligaments holding the joint together, have gotten smaller, shorter, and tighter. This is normally caused by not using our full range of motion, thanks to sitting all day in chairs with our legs together. Again, living on the floor will help immensely with opening the hips. We did not lose our hip's normal range of motion overnight, and we will not regain it quickly either. But, by applying the Yin Yoga principles to our hips, we can recover what was lost.

When we regain the range of motion in our hips, we take a big load off our knees and ankles. The hip-opening poses described in the previous section work well: Shoelace, Square, Swan, Dragons, Straddle, and Saddle poses. But, what if we have some special problems, like having had a hip replaced? Is Yin Yoga advisable in this case?

Since every body is different, every hip operation is different, as well. The surgeon is the best one to tell you what is possible for your new hip. Generally, external rotation and abduction should be no problem, but caution is needed if you are trying to adduct or internally rotate the hip. You should not be trying to recover range of motion but to thicken the ligaments and heal from the surgery. Many patients find that they automatically have a greater range of motion after surgery.

When you are given the all-clear sign from your health care team, then you can start to stress this area. Begin with an easy Deer pose, which is a gentle external and internal rotation of the hips. See how that goes before you move into deeper external rotations like Winged Dragon. Square and an easy Saddle pose may work next. Shoelace may not be a good idea because it involves bringing the knee across the midline of the body, and that is counter-indicated for hip replacement patients.

At some point, hip replacement or not, what will stop your hip movement is not going to be tension of the ligaments or muscles, but impingement of the femur in the hip socket or pinching of the buttocks between the femur and the back of the ilium. This is termed *compression*, and it is the ultimate dictator of how far we can go in any pose. Once you have reached the point of compression in your hips, you are not going to go any further in that direction for that pose. To know whether you have reached your ultimate edge, pay attention to the sensations you are experiencing. If tight muscles or ligaments are still stopping you, continue to work there—but if you feel compression you are not going get more open.

When you have reached the point of compression there is no point in trying to get more open in that direction. The shape and orientation of your bones are the ultimate determinators of how open you will get. If your knees are still up by your ears when you sit cross-legged on the floor, that may be it for you. You may never get more open than that, thanks to your bone structure. Don't let this be an excuse for not trying to get as open as you can: this is only a stopping point once you have worked through all your tensile resistance of the muscles and ligaments. But, many yoga students have severely hurt themselves by trying to push past their point of compression to get deeper into a pose than they can ultimately get. Knee damage occurs when the hips won't open any further and the students crank on the lower legs to get the foot into Lotus position. If the hips won't open, the knee twists and the pressure goes into the joint. Soon we are asking our doctor about meniscus surgery.

Pay attention: any pain is a no-no. Listen to the little tweaks your body is sending you. Little tweaks lead to big tweaks, and big tweaks lead to expensive operations.

Lower Back Disorders

In the next chapter we will take a detailed look at the spine and discover some of the benefits that Yin Yoga has for regaining the normal curve in our lower back. For now, let's look at one lower back condition that students often tell their teachers about more than any other: a bulging or herniated disc.

When we have a bulging disc (sometimes called a slipped disc, or in its extreme presentation, a herniated disc) we have compressed the front of it too often and with too great a stress. The disc is like a jelly donut: it is made of cartilage with a jelly-like center. It is designed to resist compressive stresses that would otherwise wear away the bones of the vertebrae. When we flex the spine through forward folds, we can compress the front of the disc, which forces the jelly in the middle of the disc towards the back of the disc. Over time, the jelly may start to fracture the disc and pop out, forming a little bubble.

Right behind the discs is the spinal cord. When the jelly of the disc bulges outward, it presses into the spinal cord, creating a variety of pains. Often the first sign of problem with a bulging disc occurs with a rather innocuous movement—something as simple as bending over to pick up your socks. This is the famous "last straw" effect. It is not the last movement that caused the problem; it was the years of previous repetitive stress of the disc that set you up for the injury.[3]

If you have been diagnosed with a bulging or herniated disc, you will be told to avoid flexion of the spine: this means no more forward folds. However, everyone is different. It may be possible to do flexions of the hips, as we find in Butterfly, Caterpillar, etc., without rounding the spine. Flexion of the hips can continue to work the backs of the legs, while keeping the spine straight avoids exacerbating the disc issues. Twists may also be contra-indicated at this time, depending upon how severe the disc issue is. When in doubt, leave it out. Let the body heal before you try to regain range of motion.

Sphinx pose, which is highly beneficial for students with bulging discs, is part of a sequence of restorative postures designed in the 1960s by Robin McKenzie. Basically these postures are extensions of the spine that help to push the jelly back into the donut. Stuart McGill, a professor who specializes in lower back disorders, agrees with the approach of using extensions to help with bulging discs but also requests his patients to do yang strengthening exercises to stabilize the core muscles. Postures like Crocodile or Balancing Cat, with one arm extended forward and the opposite leg stretched backward, work the back and front core muscles while—and this is the important part—keeping the lumbar spine in a neutral position.[4] Just as important as the front and back muscles are the side muscles of the core. Side Plank or side Crocodile with knees bent can strengthen the sides of the lumbar while keeping it neutral.[5]

If you have a lower back disorder, check with your doctor about what is safe to do. Let your yoga teacher know about the problem before the class starts so that you can work together to decide which poses to avoid. There are too many causes of lower back problems to allow us to investigate solutions for each situation.[6] If the problem is caused by a bulging or herniated disc, avoid flexion of the spine and deep twists. Keeping the spine straight will allow you to do many Yin Yoga poses. And extensions of the spine may be just what the doctor ordered.

Having Babies[7]

Infertility is defined as being unable to conceive after one year of trying. The cause may be the woman or the man.

Through our yoga practice we can focus on structural, hormonal, and other issues that can affect a woman's ability to conceive. Structural problems for women may include fibroids (which interfere with processes within the uterus), endometriosis, ovarian cysts, polycystic ovary syndrome (an endocrine disorder that affects approximately 5 percent of all women), vulvodynia (chronic vulvar pain with no known cause), and vaginismus (vaginal tightness).[8] Other structural problems that can interfere with conception include compression of nerves that innervate the reproductive organs. These nerves wind their way from the lumbar spine and through the inferior mesenteric ganglia. Slipped disks, derangement of the spine, and herniated disks can impinge these nerves. Alongside the nerves are the arteries that feed the pelvis and organs, which can also be compressed.

Men have similar structural issues regarding the nerves and arteries. These could include inflammation of the testes, low sperm count, and poor sperm motility.

On a hormonal basis, women who are subject to a lot of stress can reduce their fertility. This is a long-known correlation. The unfortunate part of the stress cycle is that stress interferes with conception, and not being able to conceive creates more stress! Yoga definitely helps to manage and reduce stress.

We can reduce the structural pressure on the nerves and arteries by lengthening the psoas; poses like Swan, Dragon, and Saddle are helpful. We can also look at the energy body and meridians to help bring energy to the right places. The focus here is on the heart chakra and the svadhisthana, which controls the sexual organs. Twists are great (for the heart), and Kidney work will help the second chakra, the svadhisthana. Massage of the Liver 2 and 3 points can also help with conception.[9] The Liver detoxifies the hormones and stimulates the hypothalamus. Next, work the Kidney 5 acupressure point which can assist with irregular menstruation.[10]

For the physical asanas, in a yang style, B.K.S. Iyengar has recommended flows for infertility that include Triangle, backbends, and forward bends, as well as Butterfly and Janu Sirsasana.[11] For a Yin Yoga approach, the following ninety-minute flow may be helpful. Hold each pose for three to five minutes. If you have less time, drop Happy Baby and Swan rather than shorten the amount of time in the poses. While in the postures, feel free to also reach out and apply some acupressure on the key points mentioned above.

▷ Opening meditation: focus on relaxing and becoming de-stressed

▷ Butterfly: massage the Kidney points

▷ Half Butterfly: massage the Liver points

▷ Anahatasana

▷ Sphinx and/or Seal

▷ Saddle with arms overhead

▷ Shoelace with twist

▷ Swan with psoas release (Screaming Swan option)

▷ Happy Baby

▷ Reclining Twists

▷ Shavasana

Remember, stress is a big factor in not being able to conceive, so make sure to add the ocean breath while you hold these poses. Relax, and vary the time in the poses to suit your level of practice. The intention now is to stimulate energy lines, not to be able to bring your foot behind your head. Work with attention and intention.

Pregnancy

Every body is different and what may work wonderfully for one woman's pregnancy will be ineffective for another's. Listen carefully to your body now and find out what works for you.

The suggestions in this section come from many women who shared their experiences in the YinYoga.com Forum. This is not an exhaustive investigation into prenatal yoga, and it is a very good idea to seek out a qualified prenatal yoga teacher who will teach you the basic do's and don'ts of yoga as you progress through the trimesters. As always, check with your health care provider about what you are planning to do!

Intentions are important. While you are pregnant the intention in your practice should not be to go further into poses than you have ever gone before. Range of motion is not the issue now; your baby's health and your own comfort are key. Due to the release of a hormone called relaxin, your connective tissues will start to become softer. It is easy to overstress the ligaments and cartilage in your body and possibly stretch and damage them. Whatever range of motion you had before becoming pregnant, stick with that: don't try to go further.

First Trimester

The baby is just getting nicely settled in now; generally women are told not to do inversions so that the embryo can implant firmly into the walls of the uterus. We don't have to worry too much about this in Yin Yoga because, aside from the Snail pose and Wall Arch, there are no inversions. In the first trimester the belly is not so big that it gets in the way of forward folds or twists, but you should start to reduce compression here anyway.

It is in the first trimester, and again just before delivery, that relaxin is released in high concentrations. One area that really starts to soften is the pubic symphysis, the cartilage between the pubic rami. This area will need to open to allow the baby to pass through the birth canal, but in our yoga practice we can inadvertently overstress this area. Take care in any poses involving abduction of the legs (Butterfly and Straddle) to not go further than you could go before you became pregnant.

Second and Third Trimesters

With baby growing, there is a lot of weight on the lower back. Many women crave some release in the spine and just love some nice backbends. However, lying on the belly is no longer an option and Sphinx pose, as nice as it would be, is not available … at least, not in the normal way. Now is the time to rely upon bolsters and props. Try an easy Seal or Sphinx pose with a bolster across the top of the thighs, allowing space for the belly to drop down but not press into the floor. Some women report that a block or support under the pubic bone feels better. Experiment: feel free to rest your hands or elbows on bolsters or blocks, too. The full Swan may be a nice way to get into the spine and start to work the hips, as well. Sleeping Swan can be managed by resting your upper body on a bolster.

Squat, Butterfly, and Straddle provide lots of space for your growing belly and help to keep the hips open. Just remember, don't go too far now. Just stay where it is mildly juicy. Twists are okay and can also release the spine, but due to the growing belly, we don't want to twist too deeply. Keep it in the upper chest rather than in the stomach area. Saddle is probably not a good idea right now but may be accessible if a bolster is used. Women are often advised not to lie on their backs because the weight of the baby compresses the vena cava, which is a vein that brings blood back to the heart. Shavasana now is done lying on the left side, perhaps with a bolster between the legs.

A benefit of Yin Yoga during pregnancy is the effect on the energy body of the poses. We want to stimulate the meridian lines and send Chi throughout the body and to the baby. The following flow is one way to achieve this.

▷ Opening meditation: focus on relaxing and becoming de-stressed

▷ Butterfly: works the Liver, Kidney, and Urinary Bladder lines

▷ Dragonfly (fold over the left leg, right leg, and then down the middle): works the Liver, Kidney, and Urinary Bladder lines

▷ Square pose: works the Gall Bladder and Liver lines

▷ Swan with chest up: works all six lower body meridians

▷ Seal pose: works the Urinary Bladder, Kidneys, and Stomach lines

▷ Wide-knee Child's Pose: works the Liver, Gall Bladder, and Kidney lines

▷ Easy Frog or Tadpole: works the Liver, Gall Bladder, Urinary Bladder, and Kidney lines

▷ Shavasana

Here is one woman's feedback from this flow:[12]

> I'm five months pregnant and last night I did the series of eight yin pregnancy poses Bernie suggested. Then I crawled into bed. I slept better than I have in awhile. And the ache I had been feeling in my upper back was gone. I wish I did a regular yoga routine during my first pregnancy. I'm sure I would have had a more enjoyable and comfortable experience!

As your pregnancy advances, don't hold the poses as long as you did before you were pregnant. Following are several suggestions from a Yin Yoga prenatal teacher who was eight months pregnant with twins as she related this.[13] Note her recommendation to only hold the poses for one to three minutes.

I still love practicing Yin Yoga poses, but because of the loosening in the groin's connective tissue, holding the poses for only one to three minutes now is more beneficial. Some of the poses such as Half Butterfly I will hold for five minutes, occasionally, but to be on the safe side I put a blanket under the folded leg to prevent over-stretching. In Swan, one to two minutes seems to be quite enough. I do this pose in almost every prenatal lesson, as the release on the sacroiliac joint is heavenly for most women. Due to the relaxed tissues of the pelvis, some may find it very uncomfortable.

For me, at about three months the backbending poses such as Swan and Seal became too much. Saddle with a bolster I enjoyed for longer; still one to three minutes maximum. However, from about six months onward, lying on my back for more than five minutes was very uncomfortable. A nice way to release the upper back and reduce heartburn is to stand facing a wall with your feet about two to three feet away and walk your hands up the wall. Lean into the wall to stretch your upper back and shoulders.

I found that vinyasa (a flowing yang style) practice was not suitable for me during this pregnancy; it exacerbated a lot of symptoms, including heartburn. Another thing worth mentioning is that during pregnancy my legs become stiff very easily: to avoid cramping, I try to keep the fluids moving and I rotate my ankles after coming out of yin poses, and shake them out. The yin stretches for the legs have really helped prevent stiffness. I have been focusing more on the lower body than the spine. I find yang movements, such as Cat/Cow variations work well for keeping my spine mobile.

As for forward folding and compressing the belly, as Bernie says, it will get to a point where your belly is too big to allow such a thing. I have never "hurt" myself by compressing my belly: its size means that I just can't forward fold in the same way as before: I just meet with it earlier, so taking the legs wide has become the only option.

For constipation, the Cat/Cow flow, side bends, and gentle twists work well. (A good one whilst pregnant is standing and letting your arms swing by your sides as you rotate left and right.) Twists are beneficial for the whole spine and sacroiliac joint, especially if you are having constipation; you need to be very slow and gentle. Use a bolster under the knees in the reclining twists and turn your head to the same side as your knees, rather than looking away from the legs.

Postnatal Yin Yoga

Now you have the lovely bundle of joy in your arms: time to get your body back! Roberta Hughes, an excellent pre- and post-natal Yin Yoga teacher, provides these observations:

> The six weeks following delivery is a time for healing for the mother. After delivery, most women will notice that their bodies are very stiff and tight. After I delivered, I could hardly do a forward fold. However, yin postures can be used to gently stretch the body, as well as massage the belly and stimulate abdominal muscles in a gentle way. Here is my recommendation to women who have had a healthy vaginal birth:
>
> **Week 1:** Lots of Kegel exercises and belly massage! When taking a shower, do Kegel exercises continuously as you wash and rinse your hair. Spend one to two minutes massaging the belly in a clockwise motion with moderate to deep pressure.
>
> **Week 2:** Add in forward folds to stretch the hamstrings and compress the belly. Seated forward folds such as Caterpillar and legs up the wall are perfect. Avoid hip openers and inner-thigh stretches for now.
>
> **Week 3:** Continue with forward folds. Add in reclining twists to help massage the belly, shrink the uterus, and stimulate the abdominal muscles.
>
> **Week 4:** Continue with above. Add inner thigh forward folds such as Half Butterfly and later Straddle.
>
> **Week 5:** Continue with above. Add deeper twists (seated) to work the abdominals gently.
>
> **Week 6:** After getting a check-up and clearance from your doctor, begin core strengthening work (yang) and continue with the postures above (yin).

Just one to two yin postures a day from those listed above can be very nourishing for a new mom. Practicing consistently will make a difference. Remember to be flexible with expectations, and try to feel satisfied if you only have five minutes here and there throughout the day to do yoga, rather than thirty to sixty minutes for a complete practice.

NOTES

1. Sitting on the heels is called Vajrasana; sitting between the heels is called Virasana. You don't need to do the second version; just sit on the heels.

2. The labrum is a special kind of cartilage that forms a rim around the hip socket, making the socket a bit bigger and helping to hold the femur in place.

3. Stuart McGill, author of *Lower Back Disorders* and a professor at the University of Waterloo, is often called in as an expert witness when Workers Compensation Boards refuse to pay for a back injury because the injury occurred at home. In reality, it was the nature of the job that created the condition for the injury, and not a small movement at home. In yoga classes this same error of attribution occurs: a student may hurt herself in class and blame the teacher, when it was the years of inappropriate stresses on the joints that set up the condition for the problem to occur.

4. Too often, core strengtheners end up flexing the lower back: poses like sit-ups or crunches are the worst ways to work the lower spine.

5. See *Lower Back Disorders* for a description of these exercises and many others.

6. If you have a special situation, feel free to raise it as a topic at the YinYoga.com Forum.

7. I am indebted to Nataly Pluta for much of this information. Nataly, in her workshops on fertility and yoga, cites work by Alice Domar (check out domarcenter.com.)

8. Unfortunately, not all doctors recognize these as issues and offer little help.

9. The Liver 2 acupuncture point is between the big toe and second toe, on the webbing. One inch (or finger width) above Liver 2 is the Liver 3 point. To massage these points, simply press a finger or your thumb down on the spot and massage deeply.

10. Kidney 5 is on the inner ankle, behind the medial malleolus, and one fingerwidth down.

11. Janu Sirsasana, which means "head to knee pose," is similar to Half Butterfly (one leg straight, seated forward folding posture).

12. With thanks to Sunny Mom in California.

13. With thanks to Hannah Marie from the Czech Republic.

chapter six The Physical Benefits

We have looked at *what* Yin Yoga is and *how* to practice it, and now is the time to discuss *why* we would want to do this form of practice. We will look at the benefits of Yin Yoga in three major areas: physical, energetic, and mental/emotional. There are other reasons for doing any yoga practice, such as assisting in our spiritual practice, but how yoga can assist us spiritually depends greatly on which spiritual practice we are following. Not everyone's spiritual practice is affected in the same way through yoga, but everyone can benefit physically, energetically, and mentally/emotionally.

Stressing Our Tissues

There are three things that we do physically to the tissues of our body when we stress them in yoga asana practice: compress, stretch, and twist. The results of these three stresses are called compression, tension, and shear. The drawings on the next page show the results of these stresses. In backbends we compress the facets of the vertebrae into each other (which, as we will see, is very healthy for the bones); in forward bends we stretch the fascia and muscles and stress the ligaments along the back of the spine; and in twists we provide a shearing force between the vertebrae and the ribs, which both compresses and stretches the tissues between the ribs.

The results of these stresses affect the body on many levels. Through twisting, elongating, and compressing of tissues, our bodies become rejuvenated in the same way an old sponge can be resurrected, by soaking it in warm water and twisting, squeezing, and stretching it—the old grungy particles trapped in the tissues of the sponge are released and carried away by the warm water. Similarly, our tissues are massaged by asana practice, releasing toxins and waste products. Even old scar tissue can be broken down and removed.

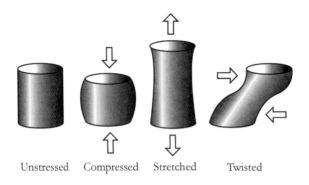

Unstressed   Compressed   Stretched   Twisted

Yoga promotes the flow of energy in the body through both stimulating energy release (especially in the active yang practices) and through removing deep blockages to the energy flow (especially in the more passive yin practices). Our blood and lymphatic fluids serve the same function as the warm water in the example of cleaning a sponge. Another metaphor is a garden hose that has been left unused for years, lying in the grass of an overgrown back yard. Insects and mud (toxins) eventually clog the hose (which could be called a meridian, or "*nadi*"). When the water (which could be called our energy, or "*prana*") is turned on, it can't flow. These clogs have to be removed, and we do so by turning on the water and bending and twisting the hose: we do yoga to the hose. Once the flow of energy has been freed or increased, nourishment flows throughout the body.

Our Tissues

Our physical bodies are made up of many types of tissues that respond differently to exercise. As we discussed in chapter 1, yang yoga is excellent at working the yang tissues, which are our muscles.[1] Yin Yoga is especially effective at working the deeper connective tissues of the body. To fully understand the physiological benefits of Yin Yoga, we need to understand the nature of these tissues.

Tissues are simply aggregations of cells in our body that have a similar purpose and arrangement. Generally, there are four main kinds of tissues:

▷ Epithelia (skin, linings of our organs, etc.)

▷ Nervous

▷ Muscle

▷ Connective (CT)

Yoga most obviously affects these last two, although it actually affects the whole body and all of our tissues. Every time we move we engage muscle to create the movement, and each movement stretches, twists, or compresses all the tissues in the area, as well as areas farther away. For our investigation of how Yin Yoga affects and benefits the physical body we will look more closely at our connective tissues. But before we head into that closer examination, it is helpful to understand one more facet of our physical body: flexibility.

The Limits of Flexibility

As we just saw, all of our physical yoga practice does one of three things to our tissues: we stretch the tissues, compress them, or apply a shear to them. This simple fact dictates what stops us from going deeper into any posture. The resistance to stretching or moving, or said another way, the limitation on our flexibility, is due to tension along the tissues, which resist further elongation, or compression, where two parts of the body come into contact and prevent further movement. If tension is stopping the movement, it is felt in the *direction away* from the movement. For example, stand up and fold one leg backward, moving your heel toward your buttock. If the heel stops before the calf presses into the back of the leg it may be due to tension in the quadriceps. This tension is in the opposite direction from the movement of the lower leg. If compression is stopping the movement, it is felt in the *direction of* the movement. In this example, compression may occur when the calf is squeezed into the back of the thigh or when the heel pushes into the buttock.

In some cases whether tension or compression is limiting movement is not easy to determine, and part of our practice is to pay attention to what is happening in the body when we move. A useful mantra to repeat during asana practice is "What is stopping me from going further?" The answer to that question may influence your practice considerably.[2]

The range of motion (ROM) we have in our joints, if it is limited by tension, can be increased through asana practice, breathing, and even diet. When the limit to the ROM has been reached and compression is stopping further movement, no amount of yoga will increase it; you have reached the limit of your ROM for that pose, in that direction. It may be possible to do a different pose to move further by going around the point of compression, but eventually, after you have worked through all the tensile resistance that you have in your tissues, what will stop you is compression.[3] However, diet, injury, surgery, and other interventions may reduce the point of compression, thus increasing ROM. For example, a woman nine months pregnant may not be able to touch her toes due to compression of her belly and legs. Yoga will not help her now! Once she has delivered her baby, the point of compression has changed, and her range of motion in that direction will increase.

When resistance (tension) limits ROM, the resistance has been found to come from four main tissues: the skin, the tendon of the muscle, the muscle itself and its fascia, and the joint capsule and its ligaments. These all provide tensile resistance to movement. The table shows how the resistance is distributed relatively in these four areas:[4]

Joint capsule and ligaments	47%
Muscle (and its fascia)	41%
Tendon	10%
Skin	2%

As shown, the biggest limit to flexibility, when it is caused by tension, is the joints' rigidity, followed by the muscle and its fascia. Yang yoga is excellent for opening us to the limits of flexibility of our muscle tissue, its fascia, and our skin. Yin Yoga is required to safely open the joints and our ligaments to their healthy limits.

Fascia

Fascia can make up 30 percent of the mass of our muscles, and for this reason muscle is more technically referred to as myofascia. The term *fascia* is a Latin word that means "band" or "bandage." Fascia, and all of its components, creates an integrating mesh that envelops our bones, muscles, and organs. Our blood vessels and nerves are held in place due to the structure and support of our fascia. For a long time, Western researchers and doctors ignored fascia and considered it merely filling for the body, of little consequence. Now we are realizing that fascia is very important for our overall health, ability to move, and proper functioning of our internal communication systems.

One map we could create for our body is that of a series of tubes within tubes within tubes, where the tubes are made of fascia. A great metaphor for understanding fascia is a package of hot dogs.[5] There is an outer plastic wrapper holding the hot dogs together: that is analogous to how our fascia wraps the muscle groups. Within this outer plastic wrapper, each individual hot dog has its own plastic bag. This is the same within our body: each major muscle group is made up of smaller groups of muscles, each with their own fascial bag. And so it goes right down to the smallest muscle fiber—all wrapped in fascia.

The Myofascia-Tendon Complex

The image shown here depicts this tubular nature of our muscle system. The outermost fascial bag is called the epimysium, which wraps the entire muscle group and gives it shape and rigidity. Without this bag, all the other tubes inside would fall apart. Inside the epimysium we have a series of parallel tubes called fascicles wrapped in their own bags of fascia called the perimysium. And inside these we have muscle fibers wrapped in a bag of fascia called the endomysium.

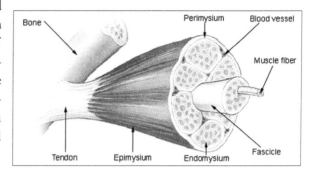

At the lower levels, the active unit of the muscle, called a sarcomere, is also encased in a fascial bag, which attaches to the fascia bag that it lies within. When the sarcomere contracts, it pulls against the fascia, which in turn pulls against the larger enveloping bags. At the level of the epimysium, the fascia becomes the tendon. There is never a sharp dividing line between one tissue and the next; rather, the fascia becomes denser and eventually becomes the tendon. In the same manner, the tendon, which joins to a bone, eventually becomes the bone.[6] This point where fascia becomes tendon is called the myotendinous (MT) junction. As the contracting force is transmitted from the sarcomere through the fascial bags, it eventually reaches the tendon, and through the tendon the contracting force reaches the bone, resulting in a movement of the bone and an articulation of a joint.

Along this chain of becoming, where the fascia becomes the tendon, which becomes the bone, there are areas that are stronger and areas that are weaker. The muscle cells are very soft and fragile, but thanks to the connective tissue covering of fascia, it is not the muscle that is damaged most frequently due to the forces of contraction or stretching. The weakest link in the chain is the MT junction. Most sports injuries occur there.[7]

If we were to take a sarcomere out of the body we would be able to stretch it about three times its resting length.[8] Inside the body, the muscle cell can normally only be stretched to about 1.5 to 1.7 times its resting length.[9] Clearly, what causes resistance to stretching our muscles is not the sarcomere itself; rather, it is the resistance of the fascia to elongation that provides the stiffness we experience in our tight muscles.

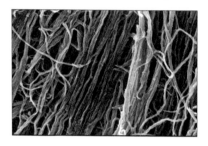

Fascia is made up of collagen, elastin, and reticular fibers. Collagen, the least elastic fiber, is one of a family of proteins, the most common of which is called type I collagen. As shown in this image, the fibers are mostly straight but they do have some sideways connecting links. The fibers are very yin-like: they resist elongation or stretching but can bend and slide along each other, which would lengthen the whole unit. If there are a lot of cross-links between the fibers, there is less ability to slide. Imagine a ladder with only one rung between the two long poles; there would not be a lot of stability. But imagine dozens of rungs between the poles of many ladders all joined together; the whole group of ladders has much more stability. It is these collagen fibers that give our fascia its ability to resist stretching.

Elastin, as the name implies, is much more elastic. Elastin fibers can be stretched up to 150 percent of their normal length without breaking.[10] Fascia has varying amounts of both collagen and elastin, which affects how flexible the fascia is. Our degree of flexibility relies upon both the number of elastin fibers we have and the organization of the collagen fibers. As we stress the fibers within the fascia a rearrangement of the collagen, their cross-links, and the elastin fibers occurs. The whole fascial bag can become permanently elongated. Within this new space, more sarcomeres will be created, normally near the MT junction.

It is beyond our scope to investigate the microscopic changes that occur as a result of stressing the myofascial-tendon complex, but it is important to note that fascia is a yin-like tissue and will respond best to yin-like stresses. A long-held static stress will help reorganize the fascia and allow it to become longer and thicker more than a short, yang-type of stress will. Sitting in Straddle fold for twenty minutes will lengthen your adductor muscles because of the effect of the stress on the fascial bags of the muscles. However, yang types of stresses are necessary in order for the muscle to become stronger. Again, balance is needed—we need both yin and yang forms of exercise to be optimally healthy.

Tendon Changing

Can we change our tendons through Yin Yoga? In the maps created by the Daoist yogis, Tendons are considered to be more than what we call tendons in the West. To the Daoists, Tendons include the muscles, fascia, nerves, and ligaments. It is easier to see how we can target Tendons, than how we can target tendons. Can we actually try to strengthen and lengthen our tendons (according to the Western definition) through yoga?

Imagine you have three elastic bands looped together to form a chain. The far right elastic is a very thick band, hard to stretch: this represents our tendons. The far left elastic is of medium thickness and can stretch, but not all that easily: this represents our myofascia. The middle elastic is shorter than the other two but very thin and very easily stretched: this represents our MT junction, the place where our myofascia become tendon. All three elastics are looped together to form one unit; now we apply a stress to the whole chain. As we pull the ends apart, the amount of stress experienced by all three elastics is the same, but the effect is quite different for each. The thickest elastic, our tendon, does not stretch at all under the stress. The medium elastic, our muscle, stretches a little. The thinnest elastic, our MT junction, stretches a lot.

If we try to increase the stress along the whole chain in order to exercise our tendon, the MT junction will stretch even further, eventually to the point of rupture. It is difficult to stress our tendons enough that a change in their microscopic structure occurs. Before that level of stress is reached the MT junction and/or the myofascia will break down. As noted earlier, the MT junction, being the weakest link in this chain, is where new tissue is added when the stress is relaxed.

When we add sarcomeres we create more strength in the myofascia-tendon complex. If we add the new sarcomere in series with the existing tissues, which means we add it to the end of the myofascia just before the MT junction, we also create more length. Through our yoga practice we create both strength and length. Body builders, who work on strength alone, tend to add new sarcomeres in parallel to the existing myofascia, thus making the muscle thicker and stronger but not longer. It is for this reason that body builders get big and cut, while yogis get long and lanky. Both become stronger but yogis get longer.

It is not really possible to target our tendons via yoga practice. Yoga will help the tendons indirectly through better blood flow, nutrition, and energy distribution but it is not practical to just try to stress a tendon. Even though tendons contribute 10 percent of the tensile resistance to our range of motion, it is an area that we really don't work on in Yin Yoga.

The Deep Fascia

The fascia that we have looked at so far was associated with our muscles, but fascia is ubiquitous and found all over the body. We have looked at one component of fascia, the fibers, but fascia also includes:

▷ Ground substances, which are extracellular fluids that create pools of watery gel through which cells can migrate.

▷ Living cells such as fibroblasts that secrete the fibers mentioned above, as well as the molecules that attract and hold water in place.

Fascia can vary in thickness and density depending on where it is and what it is being used for. Often it is found in sheets and bags, as already discussed. There is a type of fascia located just beneath the surface of the skin (called superficial fascia or hypodermis)[11] and another type directly beneath this (called deep fascia), which is usually tougher and tighter than the superficial fascia. Embedded inside this deep fascia are the tissues of the muscles, the blood vessels, and all the other tubes that wind through the body. A third kind of fascia lines the body's cavities. For our purposes we are mostly interested in the deep fascia and how it contributes to the restrictions of our range of motion.

Normal anatomy drawings rarely show the fascia and concentrate only on the muscles, leading to a misguided impression that the muscles (and the bones, blood system, and nervous system) are distinct, separate systems within our body. Distinct they are; separate they are not. Everything is interconnected, and all the tissues work together. The deep fascia merges with all the other tissues embedded within it. Even the organs cannot be completely separated from the bed of deep fascia. The organs are continuous with the fascia. We can make only an arbitrary definition as to what is muscle tissue and what is deep fascia. They are one continuum. What we do to one, we do to all.

Deep fascia:

1. Binds the muscle together, while ensuring proper alignment of the muscle fibers, blood vessels flowing through the muscles, nerves, and other components of the muscle;

2. Transmits the forces applied to the muscle evenly to all parts of the muscle;

3. Lubricates the various surfaces that need to move or slide along each other.

Fascia is not only continuous with the muscles, organs, and all tissues found within it, the fascia itself is connected together throughout the body. It is fascia that holds us together. It is fascia that keeps the bones connected and upright. Without fascia the bones would collapse to the floor like a medical school skeleton without its wires.

This continuity means a small movement in one area of the body pulls on the whole web of fascia connected throughout the body. If you are paying attention, the slightest movement at one end of the body can be felt at the other end. This is what makes it possible to feel the movement of the breath everywhere in the body—but it requires attention and practice.

Fuzz

Restrictions to our movement can come from our muscles' fascia being short and tight but fascia can restrict us in other ways too. One of the functions of fascia noted above is to allow the sliding surfaces of adjacent muscle groups to slide. If the fascia is too dry, the sliding surfaces will start to stick together. Sometimes adhesions glue the surfaces together and mobility is lost. These adhesions are made of collagen fibers that begin as thin wisps of fuzz; every night, as we sleep, our body produces fuzz between the muscle groups. In the morning, we stretch, move around, do our yoga practice—we break the fuzz. However, if we are injured, or immobilized for some reason, the fuzz doesn't get broken. Tonight we sleep again, and more fuzz is laid down upon the old fuzz. After a few days of not moving, the fuzz fibers start to intertwine and tangle and become significantly thicker. We become "fuzzed over" and our range of motion is reduced.[12]

Other injuries can also result in a reduction of our range of motion. Scar tissue can build up between the sliding surfaces of the muscles groups or in a joint capsule. No longer are we stiff and tight because of shortened muscles and tight fascia, now we have lost our flexibility due to other tissues binding us. Yoga, massage and physiotherapy are needed to reestablish our normal range of motion. We need to break down the stiff scar tissue and allow the tissues to move again.

Myofibroblasts

Sometimes, the restrictions we feel to our range of motion come from the deep fascia contracting by itself. Recently it has been discovered that fascia contains contracting elements called myofibroblasts,[13] living cells that act a bit like fibroblasts and a bit like muscle cells and contribute to wound healing. Myofibroblasts support many functions in our organs and are also found in our deep fascia. This can actually lead to problems. For example, the lumbar fascia has a high density of myofibroblasts, although the amount can vary between individuals. These contracting fibers can restrict the length of our fascia and lead to many pathologies, which in turn can lead to tissue remodeling (including shortening) and chronic instability in the lower back, headaches, and fibromyalgia. Treatments targeting the deep fascia, such as Rolfing, acupuncture, and Yin Yoga may be able to reduce the symptoms of these pathologies and correct the underlying cause.

Connective Tissues

Our joint capsules and ligaments are part of a larger group of tissues known as connective tissues (CT), a broad term that refers to biological tissues that bind, support, and protect other tissues. CT is extra-cellular, which means the tissues are not cells in themselves but are the materials surrounding and between cells. CT responds to stimuli, reacts to keep the body healthy, and creates and maintains the matrix of the body.

There are many and various cells found inside the body, as shown in the image on the next page. These include nerve cells, fat cells (adipose), blood cells (macrophages, plasma cells, mast cells, and lymphocytes), and blood vessels (capillaries). Weaving their way through all this are the fibers we have already seen, collagen and elastin, which connect the tissues.

Our connective tissue is what gives us shape and helps to restrain our movements. Bones are the most resistant to movement; cartilage is softer than bone and restrains our activities less. Ligaments, which bind bones together, also act to restrain movement depending upon their location or

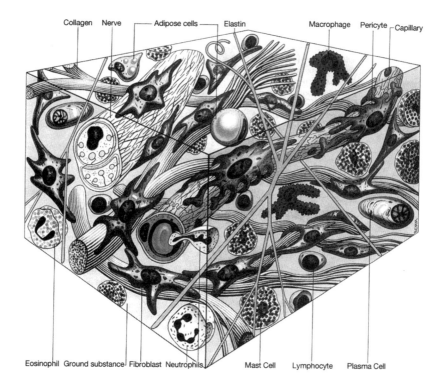

Collagen Nerve Adipose cells Elastin Macrophage Pericyte Capillary

Eosinophil Ground substance Fibroblast Neutrophils Mast Cell Lymphocyte Plasma Cell

arrangement surrounding a joint. Even less constricting than any of the above but still contributing to restriction of our activities (sometimes more than we would prefer!), fascia binds and stabilizes the body. We have already looked closely at fascia, so let's look at our other connective tissues.

Cartilage and Bones

Cartilage supports tissues and provides a degree of structure and firmness. Bones do exactly the same thing, but to a different degree. Our bones are not at all like the bones you may have seen in labs, on a skeleton, or even after a non-vegetarian meal. Usually people see or notice only the "hard" parts of a bone. This is the mineralized bone, which is generally made up of calcium salts that are deposited between the collagen fibers of the bone. What is missing is the mesh of collagen, which is much more leather-like. In living bone there is a significant portion of both collagen and calcium salts. The mineral salts help us tolerate compression of the bone while the collagen helps us resist tension that would bend or break the bone.

If the bone was made only of mineral salt and was subjected to extreme pressure, it would snap the way a dead tree branch breaks: cleanly. However, healthy, (especially young) bone, with a high degree of collagen meshing, breaks more like a living branch of a tree. If you have ever tried to snap off a living branch you know that it bends, crumpling one side while fraying the side away from the pressure.[14]

Examined closely, the inside of our bones appears porous. This sponge-like scaffolding allows the bones to be light and yet incredibly strong. The spongy-looking part is called trabecular bone. It is more elastic than the harder outer skin of the bone, which is called cortical bone. Trabecular bone is more active, more subject to bone turnover, to remodeling. The ratio of trabecular to cortical bone varies throughout the body depending upon the need. For example, the bones of the rib are not weight bearing and so they have much higher trabecular content. Our leg bones have much more cortical bone.

Cartilage is similar in makeup to bone but has a different ratio of collagen to mineral salts and other components. The cartilage in our nose, for example, has much more hydration[15] than our bones. The cartilage in our ears is even more flexible thanks to the presence of more elastin fibers. In our intervertebral disks we have fibrocartilage with a higher proportion of collagen to chondroitin. This allows the cartilage in our spines to have greater weight-bearing support than we would find in the cartilage in our ears.

Ligaments

Ligaments are similar in construction to tendons but their function is to bind bones together, usually supporting a joint. Unlike tendons, ligaments come in a variety of shapes: cords, sheets, or bands. While tendons are generally white in appearance, ligaments can be darker due to their mixture of elastic and finer fibers. Ligaments can be pliant and flexible in the directions where they are not binding the body.[16] These qualities make ligaments ideal for protecting joints, which may move in a variety of ways. Ligaments are tough, strong, and pliable, yet mostly inelastic. The iliotibial band running down the outside of your thigh, for example, is strong enough to support the weight of a car without snapping!

Not all ligaments are rigid along their lengths; some ligaments have a higher proportion of elastin than collagen. Elastin distributes stress instead of maintaining it in one place. The ligaments in the vertebral column of our lumbar spine and in our necks are especially elastic in this way. In fact, the ligaments in the lumbar spine are the most flexible ligaments in our body. When elastin fibers age they become mineralized, cross-linked with other fibers, and stiffer. When our lower back ligaments age, they become much stiffer, restraining our range of movement.

Like tendons, ligaments that are stretched suddenly and farther than about 4 percent will be damaged and tear or remain stretched.[17] In this regard ligaments and tendons are said to be plastic rather than elastic. Elastic materials, like our muscles or an elastic band, can be stretched considerably, and once stretched they will still revert back to their original shape. Plastic materials, like plasticine or our ligaments, if stretched will remain in the new shape. Once a ligament or tendon is stretched, it will not recover its original shape or size quickly. However, the body may repair it over time. For these reasons, the way in which we exercise plastic tissues must be different from the way we exercise elastic tissues. This does not mean we should not exercise our ligaments; we just have to take care so that we don't exceed their limits.

Collagen

Tendons and ligaments do not normally stretch more than 4 to 10 percent because they are made up predominantly of collagen. Collagen is a ubiquitous and amazing substance found throughout our bodies. What makes this protein so useful are its strength and resistance to stretching. Unlike most proteins, which form clumps when gathered together, collagen is fibrous and can form mats, sheets, or cord-like structures.

Collagen is what makes our teeth strong, yet it gives our skin its elasticity and strength. When it degrades it creates wrinkles. The word comes from the Greek language and means "glue producer." That gives us a sense of what it does for us; it helps hold us together.

Of the twenty-seven types of collagen, Type 1 is of the most interest in our exploration. Type 1 collagen is found in our skin, bones, ligaments, and tendons. It is found in the scar tissue that is present after healing. Collagen is what plastic surgeons use to enhance the lips of women looking for something better than what Mother Nature provided.

Fibroblasts produce collagen,[18] which is continually absorbed by the body. If the rate of production is faster than the rate of absorption, then more cross-links are created and the fibers are more resistant to stretching, but are stronger. If the opposite occurs, and the rate of absorption is faster than the rate of production, then fewer cross-links are produced and the fiber is more elastic. Researchers have speculated that exercise or mobilization could restrict the number of cross-links, thus increasing flexibility while reducing rigidity.[19] This is one model of why the practice of yoga can make us more flexible: it helps to remodel the stiffness of our collagen.

On the other hand, we do want the stability that collagen provides. As we age, or due to injury, our fascia, tendons, and ligaments, all of which are predominantly made of collagen, can get weaker. Stimulation of the fibroblasts through yoga-induced stresses can activate the fibroblasts so that they lay down more collagen, allowing our connective tissues to become stronger.

Fibroblasts create the collagen fibers found in our connective tissues, but they are not the only cells that create fibers. Other cells also create the connective tissue fibers found in our bones. In our bones, osteoblasts are also laying down fibers of collagen, which are later mineralized to create mature bone. Other cells, called "osteoclasts" do the opposite; Osteoclasts reabsorb collagen, cleaning up old bones by degrading the collagen and releasing its components into the bloodstream. Health is the balance between creation and destruction: we need to both create new, stronger tissues and clean up old, damaged ones.

Directional Stress on Connective Tissues

The direction of the collagen fibers is key. When the osteoblasts or fibroblasts create collagen fibers, they are randomly laid down in all directions. When a stress is applied along a predominant direction, electrical fields are generated by the fibers that experience the stress. This electric field prevents the osteoclasts from reabsorbing those fibers, but fibers that are not being stressed, and thus have not created an electric field, are reabsorbed. Over time, the body absorbs all fibers that are not supporting stress, leaving behind the fibers that are meant to do the work.

Astronauts in orbit live in a microgravity environment and have no stress upon the collagen fibers in their bones. Their osteoclasts are free to reabsorb their bones everywhere. Studies of cosmonauts and astronauts who spent many months on space station Mir revealed that space travelers will lose, on average, 1 to 2 percent of bone mass each month. In some astronauts the lack of stress has resulted in a much greater loss of bone density—up to 20 percent over a six-month stay in space! This loss of bone density generally occurred in the lower body and the lower back.

Connective tissues respond to demands. Stressing the body is essential in order to keep it healthy. Bones need stress to remain strong: so, too, do ligaments and fascia. Simply walking is a great way to stress the bones of the legs, pelvis, and spine. Yin Yoga is another way to provide this stress, in an intelligent and safe way, to targeted areas of the body. Specifically, Yin Yoga targets those areas where the astronauts suffered the most bone loss—the legs and lower back.

Aging or Damage of Connective Tissues

When the collagen fibers within the connective tissues are healthy they generally line up quite straight and along the direction of the predominant stress. As the body ages or is damaged, these relatively straight fibers become tangled or bent and, as a result, are shorter. These draw the muscle and bone closer together and decrease the range of motion.

Within the tangled area of the fibers, particles can become trapped. When the fibers are long and straight there is less likelihood of particles being trapped inside the fiber. What is trapped can be toxic to the body—waste products from the metabolism of nearby cells or particles of pollution from outside the body, like smoke or pesticides.

Once these particles are trapped they can remain in the body for a long time, even forever. Massage and yoga, which move the tissues of the body, can loosen up the bonds that trap these particles. Once freed, the particles can be swept into the blood system or lymphatic system and carried away, eventually eliminated from the body. Yoga stretches and compresses the collagen network of the body, which lengthens fibers and frees toxic particles.

Ground Substances and Hydration

One final topic will round out our investigation into how muscles, fascia, and other connective tissues create stability, strength, and elasticity in our body. This next topic involves ground substances, the fluids that fill the spaces between the fibers and cells in our tissues.

Imagine the inner tube of your bicycle wheel is deflated. Hold it in your hand and notice how limp and flexible it feels. You can bend it and twist it any direction you like. Now imagine it is filled with water. Feel the rigidity that has suddenly appeared. Water, which normally seems to be quite yielding, is very difficult to compress. When contained, water provides a tremendous resistance to being squeezed. Ground substances, which are sometimes called cement substances, act very much like the water in the inner tube analogy; they provide strength and support to the tissues. But they do so much more than that.

Ground substances are the non-fibrous portion of our extracellular matrix (the stuff outside the cells of our bodies) in which the other components are held in place. They are made up of various proteins, water, and glycosaminoglycans (GAGs).[20] Water can make up 60 to 70 percent of the ground substances, and it is attracted there because of the GAGs. One of the most important GAGs is hyaluronic acid (HA[21]). Various researchers have estimated that HA can attract and bind 1,000 times its volume of water.[22] Another important kind of GAG is chondroitin sulfate.

When GAGs combine with proteins they are called proteoglycans, and it is in this form that they attach to water molecules and hydrate our tissues. The proteoglycans are very malleable and move about freely. However, being made of water they also resist compression tremendously.

With water as a principal component of our ground substances, we can see why the ground substances are an excellent lubricant between fibrils, allowing them to move freely past each other. Water gives our tissues a spring-like ability, allowing them to return to their original shapes once pressure has ceased. This is crucial to our tissues' ability to withstand stresses; however, a cyclic loading and unloading of the tissue is important to maintaining health. One study found that the alteration of loading and unloading of pressure on the tissue, as long as it is not excessive, maintains cartilage health.[23]

The fluid in our joints (called synovial fluid) is also a lubricant and it too is made up substantially of GAGs. HA and two kinds of chondroitin sulfates are essential to keeping our joints working properly.

When the extracellular matrix is well hydrated, cells, nutrients, and other components of the matrix can move about freely. Toxins and waste products can migrate out of the matrix into the blood or lymphatic system to be removed from the body. The ground substances, which are also formed by the fibroblasts (remember, fibroblasts also produce collagen), are also helpful in resisting the spread of infection and are a part of our immune system barrier.

Unfortunately, as we age, the ability of the body to create HA and other GAGs diminishes. We have fewer fibroblasts available to us, and those we do have produce less HA. As a consequence, the extracellular matrix becomes filled more and more with fibers. As these fibers come closer together, they generate cross-links that bind them to each other. As a result of that, our tissues become stiffer, less elastic, and less open to the flow of the other components in our matrix. Toxins and waste products[24] become trapped in the matrix and cannot get out, and harmful bacteria can multiply freely. Immobility can also cause a steep loss in hydration: studies have shown that immobilization can cause a loss of up to 40 percent of HA, reducing the ability of our tissues to slide across each other.[25]

Fortunately exercise like yoga and massage, which stress the extracellular matrix, can help us maintain the number of fibroblasts and keep them functioning properly. This helps to keep the matrix hydrated, open, and strong.

We need these fluids everywhere in the body. The fluid of the eye is made up mostly of ground substances: this is where HA was first discovered. Our skin needs HA to remain soft. Recently cosmetic surgeons have been using HA injections, instead of collagen, as a soft tissue filler to increase the size of lips or remove skin wrinkles. The effects, however, last only six to twelve months. Chondroitin is an often-used supplement to help increase lubrication of joints. However, injections and supplements are inefficient ways to hydrate the body.[26] More effective is to coax the body to increase its own production.

Ground substances can be fluidic or gel-like, and under certain conditions they change from one to the other. When they are gel-like they provide more stability, but they are less open for the passage of materials through the matrix. When they are fluid they have less rigidity, but more openness to the flow of materials. Compression of the tissues, via yoga and other means, can temporarily transform the ground substance from gel to fluid. During the fluid state, toxins and wastes can be transported out of the matrix. Once again, we see why yoga is an excellent way to detoxify the body.

Joints

A joint is simply the joining of two or more bones. Normally, joints allow movement of the body to occur and also provide support to the body. Muscles attached to the bones via tendons provide the force or leverage to move one bone relative to another. Wrapping around the joint itself are ligaments that support and protect the joint. Inside the joints may be found synovial fluids or cartilage, or both, depending upon the type of joint and its function.

Not all joints are meant to provide large ranges of motion. Some do not allow any movement at all. There are three basic kinds of joints:

▷ Fibrous joints, where the bones are held together by connective tissues. An example of this kind of joint is the joining of the plates of our skull. No movement is desired here so the joints are fibrous, held tightly together.

▷ Cartilaginous joints, where the bones are held together by cartilage and allow slight movement. Examples of these kinds of joints are the pubic symphysis (where the two ends of the pubic bones are connected by cartilage) and between the ribs and their connection to the sternum. Slight movement is allowed in all these areas but large ranges of movement are not desirable.

▷ Synovial joints, where there is a space (the synovial cavity) between the bones. This type of joint provides the greatest degree of movement in a variety of ways.

Yoga does not try to increase the range of movement in all three kinds of joints; however, for a cartilaginous joint that has grown too tight, Yin Yoga can help to restore the normal range of motion. Yin Yoga helps rebuild the synovial joints and even extend the current range of motion.

As shown in the drawings below, there are several kinds of synovial joints in our bodies:

1. Ball and socket joints, such as the hip joint. These allow a wide range of movement.

2. Condyloid (or ellipsoid) joints, such as the knee. When the knee is extended, there is no rotation; when it is flexed, some rotation is possible.

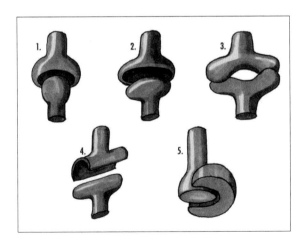

A condyloid joint is where two bones fit together with an odd shape, and one bone is concave while the other is convex. Some classifications make a distinction between condyloid and ellipsoid joints.

3. Saddle joints, such as at the thumb (between the metacarpal and carpal bones). Saddle joints, which resemble a saddle, permit the same movements as the condyloid joints.

4. Hinge joints, such as the elbow (between the humerus and the ulna). These joints act like a door hinge, allowing flexion and extension in just one plane.

5. Pivot joints, such as the elbow (between the radius and the ulna). This is where one bone rotates around another.

6. Gliding joints, such as in the carpals of the wrist. These joints allow a wide variety of movement, but not much distance (not shown here).

The Joint Capsule

The ends of the bones are coated in cartilage of varying and sometimes uneven thickness. Cartilage is softer and more pliable than the bone itself due to a higher proportion of proteoglycans to collagen. In some joints, even with the cartilage lining of the ends of the bones, the bones do not fit together snugly. In these cases, multiple folds of fibro-cartilage are employed, such as in the meniscus of the knee, to allow the bones to slide smoothly.

Around all the synovial joints is the synovium, a membrane that covers all the surfaces in the joint. The synovium forms the capsule of the joint and secretes synovial fluid into it, to keep the articulating surfaces lubricated. As we age, the synovial fluid begins to dry up. Like a leaf in autumn, we dry up and curl up, becoming more and more yin-like until we crumble into dust. This fluid (as was discussed in the section on ground substances) is made up of water-attracting molecules like hyaluronic acid and chondroitin sulfates.

A Demonstration

As we pointed out earlier, the job of our muscles is to protect the joints. The muscles do this by tightly closing the joint. There are easy ways to see this, like we described at the beginning of our journey. Again, take your right forefinger in your left hand. Relax the right hand and finger and this time apply a gentle pull with your left hand. Observe the base of the right finger ... you may notice a slight dimpling or extension across the knuckle. Even if you can't see any movement, you will definitely feel an opening there. Now contract the muscles of the right finger tightly and try to pull the finger. Notice the difference? There is no movement at all. The muscles have actively bound the joint so that no movement is possible.

The reason so much time and care is given to aligning the body and engaging our muscles properly in our active, yang-styles of yoga is to make sure the joints are not damaged by our yang movements. This is wise. As the above demonstration showed, the muscles act to protect the joint and do not allow the joint to open.

As we will soon see, however, a chronically closed area of the body, whether it is in our muscles, our fascia, or in our joints, becomes permanently closed: a process known as contracture. If we only tighten our joints and never allow them to resume their full range of movement, we will lose the original range of motion. Yang yoga is not designed to open the joints. Yin Yoga is.

Spinal Curves

The ancient Romans employed a wonderful invention in their architecture: the arch. Arches allowed stresses built up from the weight of the building materials (stones) to be distributed, which meant fewer stones were needed to support walls and domes.

Arches distribute stress, and the same principle applies to our bodies. When you look at the body you never see a straight line. Everything is curved to a greater or lesser degree. Even the longest bone, the femur, has a curve to it. Probably the most noticeable curve is the spine.

The spine has four curves. It forms a double S, with the curves in the neck and lumbar moving in opposite directions to the curves in the thorax and sacrum. The forward curve of the lumbar and cervical spine is termed lordosis. The backward curve of the thoracic spine is called kyphosis. These four curves are immensely important for an animal that walks upright; they distribute the stress of keeping the torso vertical.

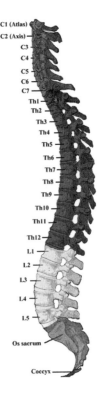

C1 (Atlas)
C2 (Axis)
C3
C4
C5
C6
C7
Th1
Th2
Th3
Th4
Th5
Th6
Th7
Th8
Th9
Th10
Th11
Th12
L1
L2
L3
L4
L5
Os sacrum
Coccyx

The spine, when healthy and possessing all its normal curves, acts like a spring. Every time we increase the pressure on our body—for example, by walking or running—the spine flexes. The curves deepen and then release. If our spine were a straight rod, the stresses would fall in between the vertebrae, and the disks cushioning the vertebrae would wear out quite quickly. Of course, the ligaments wrapping the spine also take some of the strain, but these are more responsible for taking the strain of passive activities, such as sitting or standing. Our muscles support the dynamic movement of the spine.

All forms of yoga can help strengthen the back. Yin Yoga can help reestablish the normal range of motion of the lumbar ligaments as well. But remember, everybody's bones are different. When you practice moving your spine through its full and natural ranges of motion, be aware of going too far. Be aware of pain or its precursors—small tweaks. Don't stay in a pose when the sensations of the poses are too great. The essence of the yin practice is to maintain a gentle, but persistent, pressure for a long period of time.

Other Physiological Benefits of Yin Yoga

If we consider our joints and bones for a moment, we can describe at least three big additional benefits of adding Yin Yoga to our practice:

▷ Fighting contracture of the joint capsules,

▷ Avoiding degeneration within the bones, and

▷ Reducing fixation in the joints.

Contracture

Contracture is a loss of mobility in a joint. There are many possible causes of contracture of a joint: illness, nerve damage, muscle atrophy, or problems with the cartilage or ligaments of the joint.

Everyday life can create microscopic tears in our ligaments. These small wounds are healed by the insertion of ligament tissue in between the torn edges. This function has been known for a long time; however, if the body naturally lengthens ligaments due to their constant tearing and rebuilding, why then aren't our ligaments extremely long? As Paul Grilley likes to ask, "Why don't our knuckles drag on the ground when we walk?"

University of North Carolina Professor Laurence Dahners investigated this question. What he discovered was a mechanism in which the body shrink-wraps our joints by removing materials from our ligaments. There are similar functions in many areas of our body; one part of the body creates materials (like the osteoblasts in our bones, which create bone tissue) and another part consumes or removes materials (like the osteoclasts, which dissolve bone). Health is the balance of these two functions.

An example of shrink-wrapping contracture is the classic frozen shoulder syndrome. Grandpa falls and breaks his arm, the bone is reset, and the arm rests in a sling for several weeks. When the time comes, the sling is removed, the bone has healed, but the shoulder is frozen. What happened? While there are multiple causes of frozen shoulder syndrome, such as inflammation, this cause was the lack of use of the shoulder joint. The body took away materials no longer needed, and when the time came to use the shoulder again, it couldn't respond.

The treatment for contracture is not surprising for any student of yoga: mobilization. You can do this yourself through Yin Yoga techniques and stretches, or through mechanical means. In the latter case, devices such as the Continuous Passive Motion machine move the limb through the patient's tolerable ranges of motion. This is exactly what we do in Yin Yoga: we gently but persistently move the body through its tolerable ranges of motions and hold it there. Eventually, we regain or even expand the original range of motion of the joint and combat contracture.

A study of contracture repair contrasted short, intense stresses like we find in our yang yoga practices with long-held, mild stresses like we find in our Yin Yoga practice. The researchers concluded, ". . . the longest period of low force stretch produces the greatest amount of permanent elongation, with the least amount of trauma and structural weakening of the connective tissues. Consequently, permanent elongation of connective tissue results in range of motion increases for the patient." [27] The shorter, more intense stresses were observed to have resulted in "a higher proportion of elastic response, less remodeling, and greater trauma and weakening of the tissue." [28] If our objective is to remodel our connective tissue, to fight contracture, Yin Yoga is the way to go.

Degeneration

The body continually creates and absorbs bone. If this gets out of balance we gain bone mass, causing strengthening of the bone, or we lose bone density, and the bone degenerates. Up until our mid-twenties to mid-thirties we generally gain bone mass. If we exercise conscientiously, we can continue to maintain or even add bone mass past these earlier years. Eventually, we begin to lose bone density. This condition is known as osteopenia or, in more severe cases, osteoporosis. This condition is more common in women than men, especially as women approach menopause.

One estimate suggests that 10 million Americans suffer from osteoporosis and another 34 million suffer from osteopenia, which leads to osteoporosis. Weakening in the bones results in almost 1.5 million fractures each year, with the majority occurring in the lower back. Other common sites for breakage are the wrists and hips.

Starting just before menopause, and over a four- to eight-year period thereafter, women begin to lose bone density. Osteoporosis currently affects one in four women and one in eight men. As we age, this ratio increases: by the end of menopause, 30 percent of women are osteoporotic. By the age of 80, the ratio is 70 percent.[29]

For a variety of reasons, osteoblast (bone-creating) activity may diminish or osteoclast (bone-absorption) activity may increase, causing osteoporosis. A lack of vitamin D or calcium can cause bone degeneration. Certain hormonal deficiencies such as with testosterone, estrogen, or parathyroid hormones can also contribute to bone loss. So, too, can lack of use.

Fortunately, physical activity can cause bones to grow stronger and actually change size and shape. It is well known that active people are less likely to develop osteoporosis. Autopsies have shown that attachment sites, where muscles join to the bone, grow bigger through continued use. One example is the lesser trochanter.[30] In runners this site is highly developed. Too much stress, however, can be dangerous; marathon runners have been known to develop osteoporosis later in life.[31] As in everything, balance is needed.

The bones need to be stressed to remain healthy, and the stress needs to be appropriate. Yin Yoga provides compressive stress on the bones, especially the lumbar spine. Other forms of yoga also stress the bones; most standing postures will do this. In Yin Yoga the stresses are held longer, allowing the bones more time to be stressed. This generates a larger recovery response—the bones having been stressed longer will grow stronger. Very few active yoga postures will stress the lumbar bones like Yin Yoga does.

Fixation

Ever wonder what causes all those pops and cracks you hear as you move your body? There are lots of urban myths about the cause of these, but generally, there are only three: a release of gas, friction, or fixation.

Sometimes gas bubbles will form in the synovial fluid of our joints. When these bubbles are released, a pop may happen. Other cracking sounds from the joints are caused by friction: this occurs when one part of the joint strikes another, such as when we crack our knuckles. Friction-created cracking is often heard in our knees when we lower down into a squat: this can be caused by cartilage or ligaments rubbing against each other, and sometimes is an indication of misalignment in the joint or of the ligaments.

Fixation is a temporary sticking together of two surfaces. The cracking sound is generated when the surfaces are released. That nice pop you might get in your ribs or lower back when you go into a twist is probably caused by releasing fixation. Usually it feels good because pressure has been released.

Fixation occurs under three conditions: first, the two surfaces that are getting stuck together must be smooth; second, there must be some liquid lubricant between the surfaces; third, the surfaces must be under some pressure that pushes them together.

Here's a good example of fixation: a frosty glass of ice water creates condensation (the liquid lubricant) all over the glass, including the bottom. The bottom of the glass is smooth, just like the surface of the coaster the glass is resting on. The water provides enough weight to press the glass onto the coaster. When we pick up the glass the coaster comes along with it.

This is fixation. When you pull the coaster off the bottom of the glass a sound may be audible. When you break the fixation between two bones in the body a sound may be even more noticeable. You will definitely feel the release even without the sound.

Why do we care about breaking fixation? Well, it feels good for one thing. But the main reason to break fixation is to prevent fusion of a joint.

Fusion can happen to anyone. The joint between our hip (the ilium) and our tailbone (sacrum), called the sacroiliac joint, can become fused. A 2006 study in Israel showed that 34.2 percent of men examined by computer tomography had a bridge formed between their sacrum and ilium.[32] The rate for women was far lower: 4.6 percent. This incidence of fusion, via the bridge, was age related; older subjects had a higher incidence of bridging. For some older people the joints of the lumbar spine also start to fuse.[33] Loss of flexibility here is very noticeable and a big problem.

Fusion begins with fixation, fixation is cured by mobility, and mobility of the joints is one of the big benefits of Yin Yoga.

Summary

In this chapter we have seen a variety of reasons why we would want to add Yin Yoga to our practice. This summary lists some of the main physical benefits:

▷ Improve our range of motion and flexibility.

▷ Passively lengthen our muscles through stressing the fascial bags that wrap the muscle fibers. This can be especially useful for the larger, more stubborn muscle groups such as the hamstrings and adductors.

▷ Reduce adhesions, which restrict movement between the sliding surfaces of our muscles.

▷ Stimulate growth of fibroblasts, which are the cells responsible for creating collagen, elastin, and the water-loving molecules that hydrate our tissues and joints.

▷ Make our ligaments thicker and stronger through greater collagen production.

▷ Improve lubrication through greater hydration of our tissues, which allows joints to move and fascia to slide more easily.

▷ Keep our skin younger looking through hydration, which provides room for cells to migrate through the extracellular matrix.

▷ Compress the extracellular matrix to liquefy the ground substance, which is often in a gel-like state, allowing toxins to flow out of the tissues.

▷ Stimulate the chondrocytes and osteoblasts, which create cartilage and bone, helping to reduce degeneration of these tissues.

▷ Reestablish the normal lordotic curves in the spine, specifically in the lumbar but also in the cervical spine.

▷ Prevent or reduce contracture, where the ligaments and the joint capsule shrink and reduce the joint's mobility.

▷ Reduce osteopenia and osteoporosis, which are dangerous reductions in bone density.

▷ Reduce fixation, a condition that limits the movement of our joints, and thus prevents fusion, a permanent loss of mobility in the joint.

NOTES

1. We are limiting our discussion here to the effects of Yin Yoga on our physical body, so we will be only lightly investigating the nature of our muscle tissues or the impact of yang forms of yoga on the muscles. To learn more about muscles and yoga, see Michael Alter's *The Science of Flexibility.*

2. A more general mantra useful at any time in life is a similar question, "What is stopping me?" The answer to that question is also extremely illuminating, although often very difficult to find.

3. Paul Grilley's DVD *Anatomy of Yoga* explains the concepts of tension and compression and what they mean for your yoga practice. Everyone is different: we all have different bones, joints, physiques, and life histories: there is no way everyone can look the same in every yoga pose. Understanding where your natural limits to movement are will help you avoid serious injuries in your asana practice.

4. Johns and Wright (1962): Relative importance of various tissues in joint stiffness, Journal of Applied Physiology, 17(5), 824-828.

5. Since we are all yogis now, imagine these to be tofu wieners, not all beef or pork doggies.

6. Imagine a rainbow: there is a color that is easily identifiable as red and another as yellow, but it is not possible to find the exact point where red stops and yellow begins. Red becomes yellow gradually. So it is with fascia, tendon, and bone. In our scientific methodologies we love models that cut things apart and give them discrete names, but the body is not discrete; it is an integrated whole. To describe the body, it is very useful to give names to certain parts, but never forget that the body is not merely a collection of parts.

7. Mark Lindsay, *Fascia: Clinical Applications for Health and Human Performance* (Clifton Park, NY: Delmar Cengage Learning, 2008), p. 96.

8. Laurence E. Holt, et al., *Flexibility: A Concise Guide* (Humana Press, 2008) , p. 118.

9. Alter, *Science of Flexibility*, p. 31.

10. Lindsay, *Fascia*, p. 7.

11. If you rub the skin on the back of your forearm you will notice some movement there: what allows the skin to move back and forth is the superficial fascia. Its lubricating nature allows movement between the surfaces of different tissue groups.

12. I am borrowing the term "fuzz" from Gil Hedley. The more anatomically correct term for fuzz is loose connective tissue: more correct, but not as poetic. Gil is a somanaut and can take you on a journey inside the body (the soma). His dissection labs are fascinating and highly recommended for anyone wishing to really study anatomy. You can view Gil's talk on fuzz on YouTube by searching for the "Fuzz Speech."

13. R. Schleip, et al., "Fascia is Able to Contract in a Smooth Muscle-like Manner and Thereby Influence Musculoskeletal Mechanics," *Journal of Biomechanics* 39 [2006], p. S488.

14. If this is hard to imagine, go find a green branch and try to break it cleanly. It can't be done. Only old, dried-out branches snap in half. The same difference is found in young and old bones.

15. Thanks to chondroitin sulfate, which is a water-loving molecule that holds water in our tissues.

16. Imagine a credit card: it is pliant and flexible, yet it will resist being stretched longer or wider.

17. There are exceptions, such as the ligaments in our spine, as noted earlier.

18. Fibroblasts also produce a wide variety of other substances found in the extracellular matrix, such as elastin.

19. W.M. Bryant, Wound Healing: Clincal Symposia 29(3) [1977], pp. 1-36 and R.J. Shephard, *Physiology and Biochemistry of Exercise* (New York: Praeger, 1982).

20. That's a mouthful, which is easy to gag upon when trying to pronounce. So let's just call these GAGs for short.

21. To be more current, we could call this *hyaluronan*.

22. See Eric F. Bernstein, et al., "Glycolic Acid Treatment Increases Type I Collagen mRNA and Hyaluronic Acid Content of Human Skin," *Dermatologic Surgery* Volume 27, Issue 5, pages 429–433, May 2001.

23. See "Coming Soon to a Knee Near You: Cartilage Like Your Very Own," *Science,* 5 December 2008: Vol. 322 no. 5907, pp. 1460-1461.

24. Called "*ama*" in yoga.

25. See Alter, *Science of Flexibity*, p. 54.

26. One study showed that oral ingestion of chondroitin sulfate resulted in only a 5% absorption rate, which meant that large doses were required to have any effect. Also, surgeons generally consider injection of HA directly into a joint to be a last resort, used only before surgery may be required.

27. George R. Hepburn, "Contracture and Stiff Joint Management with Dynasplint," *Journal of Orthopaedic & Sports Physical Therapy* 8:10 [April 1987], pp. 498-504.

28. The elastic response occurs when the tissues return to the original lengths.

29. L.J. Melton, 3rd "How many women have osteoporosis now?" *Journal of Bone Mineral Research* 10 [1995], pp. 175-77.

30. An attachment site of the hip flexor muscles on the inner femur.

31. See arthritis.org for more on the risks of running.

32. Gali Dar and Israel Hershkovitz, "Sacroiliac Joint Bridging: Simple and Reliable Criteria for Sexing the Skeleton", *Journal of Forensic Science* 51 [2006], pp. 480-83.

33. Sometimes with degenerative joints, a procedure called arthrodesis is used to deliberately fix joints, to force them to fuse together.

chapter seven The Energetic Benefits

We have been looking at the physical benefits of Yin Yoga from a Western point of view, but there are many potential models we can use to explain what happens as we practice yoga. The Western viewpoint, that of modern medicine and science, is particularly good for examining our physiology, but when we start to examine what happens inside our body from an energetic point of view, other models can be just as useful. In this chapter we will contrast three separate models: that of the Indian yogis, that of the Daoists, and that of Western science. The benefits we can obtain from our yoga practice are quite varied and depend upon our initial intentions.

A Yogic View

In India the practice called yoga evolved over thousands of years. The intentions of the practice of yoga were varied; there never was one yoga. There is no yoga tree that shows the evolution of all the various forms of yoga we know today. Rather, there is a forest called yoga, within which many wondrous and frightening forms of practice have existed. There are dozens of definitions of the word *yoga*. At times *yoga* meant to hook up your chariot, upon your death on the battlefield, and rise up and pierce the disc of the sun, thus becoming immortal. Many yogis were feared as magicians who could take over the bodies of the dead and bring them back to life. Other yogas allowed the yogi to fly through the air, split into many bodies at once, enter another living body, and take control. Parents would frighten their children into obedience by warning them that the yogi would come and eat them if they misbehaved: this was not quite an idle threat because some yogis did kill and eat people. Some yogis were mercenaries, feared warriors with weapons unknown in the West, such as the deadly flying discs. A yogi could come into a man's home, take any food he pleased, take pleasure with the man's wife, and leave with money or jewels and suffer no rebuke or interference from the owner of the house.[1]

These yoga practices are obviously quite different from what we think of as contemporary yoga. Today, yoga is thought to be sweet, pure, and practiced with intentions of health and spiritual progress. And these forms of yoga did and do exist in the yoga forest, but these were not the only trees in that mysterious land.

Around 200 C.E. a classical form of yoga was blossoming, summarized succinctly by a text known as the Yoga Sutra.[2] In this school of yoga, a yogi practiced to master his mind and still the whirling thought-forms fluctuating within. Once the mind was tamed, the yogi was able to enter a state of deep meditative absorption known as samadhi. The intention of this particular practice was to obtain liberation from the bonds of matter and, after leaving the body, become liberated. Only after death could liberation be achieved.[3] The body and mind were the enemy, formed of *prakriti*—created matter and energy, which entraps us and deludes us into thinking that we are our bodies or that we are our minds.[4] Our true substance, called *purusha*, is pure consciousness: the witness. Nature entraps consciousness, and, thus, nature was our enemy. This fierce yoga of strict asceticism and meditation was not for everybody, and not all agreed that the mind and body were the enemy.

A new form of yoga grew in the forest as a reaction or counterpoint to classical Yoga's life-denying practices: Tantra. Tantra Yoga embraced life: one could only become liberated if one had a body. To become liberated while alive, to become a *jivan-mukta*, required that we transform our body and channel our inner energies. Tantra created a sophisticated model of these inner energies, also called subtle energies because it is not easy to discern them, let alone master them. A later offshoot of Tantra Yoga, called Hatha Yoga (which we discussed briefly in chapter one) maintained the subtle body model created by the Tantrikas but dropped much of the more esoteric and socially unacceptable Tantra practices. With Tantra and Hatha, yogis now were practicing to enhance health and make the body stronger, rather than to starve the body and die to this squalid existence. A key to the managing of our subtle energies was the practice of pranayama; the management of our life force, known as prana.

Prana

The psycho-spiritual science[5] of *pranayama* developed around the concepts of energy (*prana*), the little rivers of energy flowing within our bodies (*nadis*), and the major energy plexuses (*chakras*). A Western definition of *energy* is the ability to do work. An Eastern explanation is not so different; energy allows us to be, live, and act in the world. Just as we use the term *energy* to denote all the various kinds of energies that exist, so, too, in the yogic models one term is used to encapsulate all of the various kinds of energies: *prana*.

Prana is life and is also often considered to be our breath. It literally means, "breathing forth." This understanding is not unique to India. Many ancient cultures equated life and breath. In Latin, the word *spiritus* also means breath. In the Rig Veda, the oldest Hindu text, prana is claimed to be the breath of the cosmic purusha.[6] *Prana* is an overarching term with many subcategories.

An understanding of prana is important for the yogi. The control of our energies, our prana, allows us to maintain or improve our health, to provide the energy needed to delve deeper into the mysteries of our existence, and to calm the inner winds that blow our minds from one thought to another. Yin Yoga helps us to manage our pranic energies in several ways, as described in chapter 2.

Learning how prana works and how to free this energy is part of the psycho-spiritual practice known as pranayama. The word *pranayama* is really two Sanskrit words: *prana* and *ayama*. This is often misunderstood, and many students think the two words are *prana* and *yama*. *Yama* means to restrain or control, *ayama* means to not do that. Thus in a pranayama practice we are trying to free up the energy of prana, not restrain it. This can be confusing, as many teachers and authors prefer to interpret pranayama as controlling the breath. Perhaps a better way to think of pranayama is to consider it regulating the breath, but in such a way that the prana is actually freed or extended in a controlled way.

Why would we want to regulate the breath? If you have ever attempted to meditate and still the turnings of your mind, you know how difficult this is. Zen is one discipline that attempts to still the mind through sheer willpower. This is a very difficult practice, and it is not surprising that Zen was the way of the samurai. Yogis sought an easier route to the same goal, through regulating the breath. If the breath is quiet, the mind is still.

Inside the body there are five major and five minor kinds of prana.[7] We will look only at the major forms:

1. *Prana*: the upward lifting energy. This can be confusing; the prana vayu is a subset of the overall term for all energies, also called prana.[8] The prana vayu is responsible for the energy of the heart and the breath. When we see a tree's branches reaching upward to the sun, that is prana energy being expressed. When we feel our inhalations lift our spirit, along with our shoulders, that is prana. Try this: stand in Mountain Pose—tune into your prana as you inhale and raise your arms overhead: feel the lifting energy as your arms ascend.

2. *Apana*: the downward, rooting energy. The apana vayu is responsible for elimination, both through the lungs (carbon dioxide) and the digestive tracts. The roots of a tree searching downward for stability are expressing apana. The rooting downward of our exhalations tap into the same energy. We can tune into apana while in Mountain Pose and after we have raised our arms overhead: now start to bring the hands down to the chest; feel the rooting energy as your arms descend.

3. *Samana*: the balancing energy. The samana vayu is responsible for digestion and the metabolism of our cells. Its direction is inward. We can tune into samana when we draw our arms inward: stand in Warrior 2 with your arms apart—as you exhale draw your hands to your heart and feel the energy of hugging our muscles into our core.

4. *Vyana*: the outward-moving energy. The vyana vayu is responsible for the movement of our muscles and for balancing the energy flow throughout our body. We can tune into vyana when we extend our arms out as we do in Warrior 2 pose: feel the outward-moving energy as you extend your limbs.[9]

5. *Udana*: the "up breath" or upward-moving energy. The udana vayu is responsible for producing sounds and is the energy of the five senses. Some texts place this only in the throat but other texts say that it circulates in all the limbs and joints.

None of these energies exist in isolation. Sensing the flow of energy is a meditation practice all on its own. Just sitting for a few minutes watching the prana and the apana requires attention. As we hold our Yin Yoga poses for five minutes or longer, we are given the opportunity to practice this meditation on energy. As a result of this inner awareness, our thoughts will slow down just as the sutras promise.

Energy does not simply exist; it flows. Just as a garden hose channels water, as our nerves channel electrical energy, and as our blood vessels channel chemical energy, so, too, is prana channeled in our bodies. These channels are known as nadis.

The Nadis

Water requires banks before it can become a river; prana also requires a path along which to travel. These pathways are the *nadis*, which means "little rivers." Some ancient texts, such as the Shiva-Samhita, claim there are 350,000 nadis. Many texts claim there are 72,000. The Tri-Shikhi-Braha-mana Upanishad tells us that the number is countless.

Despite the large number of nadis detected by the yogic sages, usually only eleven or twelve are named, and of these only three are really discussed. However, even here the texts vary considerably in the descriptions of each nadi.[10]

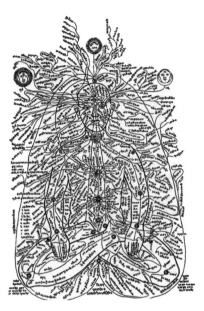

The Nadis as depicted by the Tibetan sage, Ratnasara

The three nadis of most importance are:

▷ The *sushumna* nadi

▷ The *ida* nadi

▷ The *pingala* nadi

The Sushumna Nadi

This is the most important nadi. Most texts agree that this channel begins in the muladhara chakra, which is located at the base of the spine. The channel corresponds to the Governor Vessel meridian in the Daoist view of energy flow. The sushumna flows inside the core of the spine, but it is not the spine; it is subtler than that. The perceived function of the sushumna depends upon the school of yoga one is studying.

In Tantra and Kundalini Yoga, and in many Hatha Yoga schools, the sushumna is the key channel within which *kundalini* energy flows. Kundalini is said to be a special form of energy or the highest form of prana. The term refers to the power of the snake, which is envisioned to lie coiled up at the base of the spine, dormant and awaiting awakening. In some schools the kundalini energy is known as shakti.

Georg Feuerstein suggests that prana may be considered like the energy in an atomic bomb, while kundalini energy is like that of a hydrogen bomb.[11] Shakti energy is directed upward from its home just below the *muladhara* chakra toward the *ajna* chakra (according to Dr. Motoyama) or the *sahasrara* (according to Georg Feuerstein). The intention is to bring kundalini up the sushumna to the top of the head where Shiva awaits reunion with Shakti.

Once the kundalini has been awakened and raised up the sushumna to the top of the head, many psychic phenomena may occur. Inner sounds, special sight, and insights can be perceived. *Vibhutis*[12] such as clairvoyance, telekinesis, telepresence, and telepathy may be manifested. Jivan-mukti (liberation while still residing in the body) is achieved in this manner.

The Ida and Pingala Nadis

Running alongside the sushumna nadi, on either side of the spine, are the *ida* and *pingala* nadis. Ida refers to the *chandra* (yin) energies of the moon, while pingala refers to the *surya* (yang) energies of the sun.[13]

The flow of these two channels is disputed. Modern teachers generally teach that the ida begins in the muladhara at the base of the spine and rises up the left side of the spine until it reaches a chakra. It switches sides at each chakra until it reaches the back of the head. Climbing over the head, it comes down the forehead until it ends in the left nostril. The pingala runs similarly but begins on the right side and ends in the right nostril. Together they form a caduceus, two snakes spiraling their way around the sushumna nadi.

Dr. Motoyama's research reveals that none of the yogic texts actually describe in detail the paths of the ida and pingala. There is certainly no discussion of the nadis crossing at the chakras. Implied is that the nadis flow up alongside the spine much like the Urinary Bladder lines in Chinese medicine.

An interesting thing happens to the flow of energy in our ida and pingala channels: about once every ninety minutes or so, our breath switches sides. See if you can tell which nostril is more open right now. When we are healthy, the breath switches nostrils every ninety minutes or so. When we are ill, this happens maybe every few hours. It has been said that when death is near, the breath does not switch nostrils at all.

When the breath is flowing out of the surya (the right) nostril, we are in a yang, energized state. When the breath is flowing out of the chandra (the left) nostril, we are in a yin, passive state. There are several forms of pranayama that help to balance the surya and chandra energies, such as Nadi Shodana (described in chapter 2). These practices are normally done after asana practice, but they can be added to seated Yin Yoga poses.

According to many teachers, there are certain activities that must be abstained from if the wrong nostril is open. For example, Pattabhi Jois, in the book *Yoga Mala,* warns that one must not make love when the sun is shining, or when the right nostril is open. When the right nostril is open, it is the same as the sun shining.[14]

Chakras

Within the human body there are almost 100 plexuses. A plexus is a joining together (as opposed to a branching apart) of nerves forming a nerve net. The best known is the solar plexus, which is an autonomous cluster of nerve cells behind the stomach and below the diaphragm. Some scientists call the solar plexus our second brain. Blood vessels can form plexuses, such as the choroid plexus in the brain. And yogic sages tell us that nadis also form a network creating plexuses, which they call *"chakras."* Chakras are wheels or circles and are models of the way the subtle energy in our bodies can be networked into gathering points, in the same way nervous energy may be networked in our solar plexus.

Buddhist yogis developed one of the earliest models of the chakras 1,500 years ago. They helped develop the Tantra school of yoga. Their map showed five chakras, one for each of the meditation Buddhas. In the Tantra school of yoga, as practiced in India by Hindu yogis, seven major plexuses were detected, one for each heavenly plane of existence (or *lokahs*), ranging from the earth to the highest heaven.[15]

The theories of chakras are varied and diverse. There is no consensus on the number of chakras we have (some texts describe twelve or more), their location, descriptions, or even the purpose or function of them. Often chakras are depicted in diagrams as having a certain number of lotus petals, a particular color, sound, and symbol. But here, too, there is a wide diversity. What is commonly agreed is that the chakras are energy centers of the subtle body.

Chakra is not another term for the nerve plexuses or endocrine glands of the physical body, even though they may reside in the same general location. Similarly, chakras are not physical organs of the body. Much has been made of the close proximity and similar functions of the chakras and the endocrine organs. However, the yogic texts do not make such claims, and it has been only in the last few decades that some teachers have made this association.

There are many books available today that describe chakras in detail.[16] It is difficult to find a definitive explanation of what chakras are supposed to do, but it is safe to say that a chakra is a center of subtle energy (prana or kundalini) that needs to be manipulated in order to achieve complete physical and spiritual health, and eventual enlightenment. In ordinary individuals, the chakras are undeveloped or even dormant. The practice of yoga helps to awaken the chakras, allowing prana to flow through them. Eventually, when all six of the lowest chakras have been opened, energy is free (*ayama*) to reach the highest chakra, and liberation is possible.

Dr. Motoyama's View

One of the purposes of Tantra and Hatha Yogas is the gradual cleansing and opening of each chakra. Once these energies' vortexes are open, the flow of kundalini, or shakti energy, can rise up the central channel and consciousness merges with God. The impression is easily gained that these chakras must be opened sequentially, beginning with the lowest and moving upward. This is not actually stated in any of the ancient texts on yoga. Many people may have one or two chakras already open but have lower ones blocked.

In Dr. Motoyama's experience the chakras should be opened in a specific sequence but not starting from the bottom one, the muladhara.[17] He strongly advises the student begin with the ajna, which is between the eyes. He says, "… if the ajna is awakened first, the overpowering and potentially dangerous karmic forces hidden in the lower chakras may be safely controlled." After awakening the ajna, the yogi then opens the muladhara and then the second chakra, the svadhisthana, and then on up the line.

Through his clairvoyant visions, Dr. Motoyama reports that chakras are less like wheels and more like cones, with the root of the cone in the spine and the top, open end of the cone on the front surface of the body. He calls the front of the chakra the receptor.

There is another major difference between Dr. Motoyama's view of the function of the chakras and those of most authors on yoga: Dr. Motoyama has determined that the chakras are bridges between three bodies we each possess. These three bodies are:

▷ The physical body and its mind: the consciousness associated with the physical.

▷ The astral or subtle body and its mind: the consciousness associated with emotion. This is the home of prana or Chi. It is interesting to note that Chi obeys physical laws because it bridges both the physical and the astral bodies. Like the beam of a flashlight, Chi weakens over space and time.

▷ The causal body and its mind: the consciousness associated with wisdom and intellect. This is the home of a higher psychic energy Dr. Motoyama calls *"Psi."* It is also interesting to note that physical laws do not bind Psi because Psi does not touch the physical body. It does not weaken over space and time, but like a laser stays powerfully focused wherever it is directed.

Dr. Motoyama tells us that the physical body is yang compared to the yin nature of the astral and causal bodies. It is the chakras that link these bodies together and allow information and energy to flow between them. It is due to this linkage that yogis throughout the ages have been able to perform normally impossible feats. For example, a master buried alive for weeks with no air, food, or water survives because of his ability to transform astral energies into physical energy.

The Benefits of Pranayama

The yogis of India were primarily interested in spiritual liberation, either while alive in this body (Tantra Yoga) or in a disembodied state after death (classical Yoga). To achieve this liberation, the Tantric or Hatha Yoga traditions required cleansing and opening the major pathways, the nadis, and stimulating the flow of prana through them. The breath was the main tool used to stimulate the energy flow, while the physical practice of Hatha Yoga became the main tool used to dislodge any blockages to the flow of prana.

There are two key reasons for doing yoga, from an energetic perspective: the first is to stimulate or turn on the energy flow and the second is to remove blockages.[18] This is analogous to a garden hose that has been left abandoned in a back yard for many years. Over time, mud and insect debris clog the hose. When we go to use the hose again and first turn on the water (which is analogous to stimulating the flow of prana) nothing happens. We have to do some yoga to the hose: we bend it and twist it to loosen up the blockages, turn on the water, and now the energy is free to flow. This is what we do in our yoga practice: we move the body via our asana practice and turn on the energy via our breath.

There are many forms of pranayamas that are taught by the masters, and these can be dangerous to play around with.[19] Like any tool, pranayama can be mishandled: the guidance of an experienced master is essential if we wish to explore the more esoteric pranayamas, especially the very yang-like versions. However, the more yin-like breath work as described in chapter 2 can provide a large measure of the benefits the yogis sought: a calm mind.

A Daoist View

In the first chapter, we began to look at a Daoist map that described the experience of the yogis of ancient China. We saw how, of the five major Daoist practices, inner alchemy became the practice of choice for the yogis seeking physical immortality.[20] A major component of the Daoist practice was controlling energy, just as it was in India. While the intentions were similar, the processes were different, and the maps created by the Daoists display different concepts and practices. In time, the maps blazed by the early Daoists became useful to doctors trying to treat their patients and a branch of medicine evolved, which today we call Traditional Chinese Medicine.[21] Key to understanding Chinese medicine and the inner alchemical practices of the Daoist (and to understanding the benefits for us modern yinsters) is to be familiar with the important concepts found in the Daoist maps.

Chi

In Chinese medicine, a model of the body is used that is based upon energy and the passages along which energy flows to nourish the organs. Just as prana has many forms, there are three major energies in the Chinese model: *Chi* (also spelled *Qi*), *Jing* (also spelled *Ching*), and *Shen*. These passages, similar to the yogic nadis, are called meridians.[22] And where the yogic models include psycho-energetic centers, the chakras, in the Chinese models the organs are the important centers for energy storage and distribution. In the Chinese model, the organs are actually functions residing not just within the physical location of the organs as we know them in the West—but within every cell of the body.

Chi is derived from the word *breath*, just like *prana* or *spirit*, and denotes this essential life force. Unlike prana, Chi is a much broader concept. It is not just life force: Chi is the mystical, subtle force that moves the universe. One meaning for the word is "weather." Another is "heaven's breath." Chi is the pulsation of the universe itself. It is found everywhere, in all things animate and inanimate. It is not quite energy or matter; rather, it can be considered energy on the verge of becoming matter, or matter on the verge of becoming energy. Chi is becoming and being. Chi doesn't cause things to happen, as Chi is always present before, during, and after any change or event.[23] Whether Chi is real or merely a metaphor is not important: thousands of years of successful medical use show how useful this map is.

When we looked at the Indian view of energy, we noticed that there were five main kinds of prana within the body. In a similar manner, the Daoist yogis and doctors discerned five kinds of Chi, known as the fundamental textures. These are:

▷ Chi

▷ Blood

▷ Jing

▷ Shen

▷ Fluids

Blood

Blood is what we would normally think of as blood in the West but with a bit more to it. Blood moves constantly throughout the body, flowing in both the blood vessels we are familiar with in the West and also through the meridians. Blood nurtures, nourishes, and moistens. Blood is a yin complement to the yang Chi. Where Chi excites, Blood calms. Where Chi advances, Blood remains.

Jing

There are many interpretations of what exactly Jing is and does. Sometimes referred to as *essence*, Jing can be considered the material basis of our body that nourishes and fuels our cells. Jing also cools the body and thus is yin in nature. Jing controls the long-term cycles of life, rather than the quick daily rhythms. With an ample supply of Jing, we grow wiser as we mature in old age: without enough Jing our aging is less graceful and we rage against the changes in our body.

One definition of *Jing* notes that it is a form of Chi found in sexual fluids. Another possible consideration is that Jing is the carrier of our original physical nature. It is in the DNA that our cells build upon. Jing is stored in the kidneys and is carried in the semen and menstrual fluids. From the Kidneys, Jing is distributed to all other organs to help them in their normal, healthy functioning.

There are two kinds of Jing: "before-heaven"—the Jing that is given to us before our birth—and "after-heaven"—the Jing that we gain from living, eating, and exercising. Unfortunately, our store of the prenatal Jing is fixed and cannot be replenished. Once it is used up, life is over. Jing is consumed constantly by just being alive; however, some activities consume Jing too quickly: stress, illness, too much sex or improper sex, or abuse of substances. Some activities restore Jing, but only the postnatal kind.

Think of Jing as two bank accounts: one is a savings account into which you can never put more money. This account is filled at birth. The second account is a checking account, from which money can be withdrawn and deposited. When your checking account is overdrawn, funds are automatically transferred from your savings account. Once your savings account balance reaches zero, tilt! Game over.

The secret to longevity is to use up as little before-heaven Jing as possible while building up a store of after-heaven Jing through Daoist practices such as Chi-gong, Tai Chi, or Yin Yoga. Beyond these practices, just living mindfully will lengthen your life and develop wisdom: eat healthy foods, get plenty of sleep, hang out with inspiring people, and avoid unhealthy activities, individuals, and practices. [24]

Shen

Shen is a broad term. A poor English translation would be *soul*. Sometimes *Shen* is used as the word for *God* by Chinese Christians. It is the opposite density from Jing; Shen is the most refined and subtle form of Chi. Shen is the inner strength underlying Chi and Jing, and is closely associated with consciousness. Shen is awareness. It is also associated with creativity. If Shen is weakened, a person will suffer in many ways; forgetfulness and foggy thinking, insomnia, or erratic behaviors may arise.[25]

Fluids

Fluids are all the other liquids we have not yet discussed. These include saliva, urine, perspiration, and all the digestive liquids. Some Fluids are dark and heavy, while others are light and clear. Fluids lubricate and nourish, feeding the skin, hair, muscles, joints, brain, organs, bones, and marrow. While related to Blood, these other Fluids are not as deep or as important as Blood.

Other Forms of Chi

The above categorization of Chi is not the only model used. Some Chinese practitioners have different mappings for Chi. Just as the yogis in India discovered 10 kinds of prana, some Daoist yogis have discovered 32 different types of Chi. Chi has been categorized as:

▷ Yuan Chi—Original Chi given before birth, which governs our zang/fu organs.

▷ Gu Chi—Chi from food, also called Grain Chi

▷ Kong Chi—Chi from air.

▷ Zong Chi—Gathering Chi created by combining Gu Chi and Kong Chi. Zong Chi circulates the blood.

▷ Zheng Chi—True Chi created from Zong Chi when it is acted on by Yuan Chi. This is the Chi most often referred to in texts.

▷ Ying Chi—Nourishing Chi, which nourishes the organs and produces blood.

▷ Wei Chi—Defensive Chi, which protects and warms the body.

▷ Organ Chi—Each organ has its own form of Chi.

▷ Earth Chi—This form is often the main concern of Feng-Shui, the art of arrangement your home in accordance to the flow of Chi in nature.

▷ Sun or Sky Chi—the energy we receive from above.

This is not a complete list. Many of the above forms of Chi combine to create different types of Chi. Like Jing, a certain amount of Chi is given to us before our birth but we can also gain more Chi through our diet, breath, exercise, and meditation.

Function of Chi

One very important purpose of Chi is to support the function of the organs. Chi helps to digest food and transform it into blood and energy. Chi defends the body against infection and pathogens. Chi also maintains the body's temperature and circulation; it keeps the organs in place, keeps the blood in its vessels, and governs elimination of excess materials. Chi makes all movement and growth possible. When Chi is out of balance it can become deficient or stagnant; these are opportunities for disease and illness to arise.

There are four key pathological conditions of Chi:

▷ Deficient Chi: manifests as shortness of breath, dizziness, fatigue, paleness

▷ Sinking Chi: manifests as prolapse of the organs

▷ Stagnant Chi: manifests as various forms of pain

▷ Rebellious Chi: manifests as coughing, belching, vomiting, or hiccupping.

It is clear how important Chi is to our health. From a purely pragmatic perspective, learning to acquire and utilize Chi properly, to keep it strong and mobile, will assist in extending a person's lifespan. The quality of that life depends upon other aspects of Chi, as well: the strength of the Shen (spirit) energy and the health of the organs.

To lay out the full extent of the maps that the Daoists created for energy would take several volumes. We will suspend our investigation into the Daoist concept of energy and move now to look at the next important concept, the Organs. Unlike the concept of chakras developed by Indian yogis, which are found in the subtle body, Organs are physical.

The Organs

In the Daoist concept of Organs, they are not merely physical entities; they are functions. These functions reside throughout the body, not in one place. Just as the body overall needs these functions to maintain health, each cell also requires the same functions. We cannot say that just the body needs oxygen and needs to eliminate wastes. The function of respiration (via the Lungs) and elimination (via the Kidneys) are pervasive: every cell in our body needs to be fed, nourished, and have its waste taken away.

As we have already noted, Chinese medical models often refer to the Organs with a capital letter to differentiate their model from the Western view of organs, which are denoted by a lowercase letter. When you see the word Heart, you will know you are dealing with the function of the Heart Organ, rather than the physical heart organ, as we know it in the West.

The functions of the body are based upon the five solid Organs, referred to as the *zang* organs. These are the Heart, Spleen, Lungs, Kidneys, and Liver. Everything in life requires yin and yang for balance; thus these solid,

ORGAN	TYPE	PAIRED	EMOTION	ELEMENT	FUNCTION
Stomach	Fu	Spleen	Worry/ Creativity	Earth	Reservoir for food and water
Spleen	Zang	Stomach		Earth	Controls digestion, stores intention or determination
Liver	Zang	Gall Bladder	Anger/ Kindness	Wood	Stores blood, regulates Chi flow, controls tendons, seat of Shen
Kidney	Zang	Urinary Bladder	Fear/ Wisdom	Water	Regulates water volume, coordinates respiration, stores Jing
Urinary Bladder	Fu	Kidney		Water	Storing and discharging
Gall Bladder	Fu	Liver		Wood	Reservoir for bile (Liver Chi)
Heart	Zang	Small Intestine	Fright/ Love	Fire	Blood circulation, mental functions
Lungs	Zang	Large Intestine	Sadness/ Beauty	Metal	Controls Chi and respiration, regulates water flow
Small Intestines	Fu	Heart		Fire	Receives and contains food and water
Large Intestines	Fu	Lungs		Metal	Involved with transport and transformation
San Jiao	Fu				Digestion
Pericardium					Circulation

yin-like zang Organs have their yang counterparts in the hollow *fu* Organs of the Urinary Bladder, Gall Bladder, Small Intestines, Stomach, and Large Intestines. Each pair of Organs is connected via meridian channels. Each of the zang Organs is also associated with one of the five elements of Daoist cosmology and, through these elements, our emotions.

Zang Organs

These are the viscera of the body, the solid organs that store our energies and fluids. These Organs can be considered yin relative to their partner fu Organs because they are solid. The zang Organs regulate.

The Heart (and pericardium)

The Heart is the ruler of all the zang Organs. The Heart controls our mental activities and the circulation of blood. Problems with the Heart are often seen in the face, complexion, and tongue. In this model, it is not the brain that controls our thoughts. The brain is simply the place where thoughts are received and stored. Our mental health, our ability to think, and the vigor of our blood are directly related to the strength of the Chi in our Heart. Weak Chi here can result in insomnia and poor sleep, disturbing dreams, dullness, and heart palpitations. If the Heart is weak we may be easily startled or frightened; if the Heart is strong we can easily feel love. Feeling love and feeling loved can strengthen the heart.

The Spleen

In Chinese medicine, the Spleen is essential to the process of digestion and distribution of nourishment. If the Spleen's Chi is strong, the food's essence is spread throughout the body. If the Chi is weak, the body becomes undernourished and weak. This same distribution occurs for water, too; the Spleen ensures proper hydration of our cells and the elimination of water through the kidneys. Because our blood is mostly water, the Spleen directly affects the quality of our blood. The Spleen also controls the proper functioning of our limbs and maintenance of our skeletal muscles. The Spleen affects our mental function, especially our intention, willpower, and awareness of possibilities for change.

Weakness in the Spleen can often be seen in the lips and mouth. If things taste good, the Spleen is working well. If the Spleen Chi is weak, worry may be a constant companion. Worry can weaken the Spleen (and also create stomach problems.)[26] If the Spleen is strong, we find great stores of creativity.

The Lungs

The Lungs control Chi (breath), and since this is the first contact with the external winds, the Lungs have to be vigilant. They are associated with Defensive Chi to ensure nothing harmful enters the body. The Lungs help to control water and fluids. Edema (water retention) may be caused by a weakness in the Lungs.

The quality of Lung Chi is often seen in the skin and hair. Sadness that won't go away may be a sign of weakness in the Lungs. A lot of grief and sadness can weaken the lungs: just note what happens when we are sad and cry—the lungs involuntarily spasm. Our ability to see and appreciate beauty indicates health of the Lungs. Noticing and enjoying beauty can strengthen our lungs.

The Kidneys

The Kidneys store Jing. Here this essence of our body can be converted into Kidney Chi, which is used to help the Kidneys control water. The Kidneys send clear, healthy water upward to circulate in the body and used, turbid waters downward for elimination. The Kidneys also govern utilization of water. Because blood and bones are so intimately connected to water, the Kidneys are also responsible for their proper functioning. Determination is said to be stored in the Kidneys, which are also directly connected to reproductive health and function.

Problems with the Kidneys can be seen in the ears and genitals. Problems may result in anxiety or emotions of fear arising at inappropriate times.[27] Too much fear can weaken our Kidneys, but they can also be the source of deep wisdom: when the Kidneys work well, we mature gracefully.

The Liver

The Liver is the home of Shen, the soul. When our Shen is calm the Liver is functioning well, and we can watch the world unfold dispassionately. The Liver has many physiological functions, but mostly it regulates the amount of blood in circulation. While the Heart may govern the flow of blood, the Liver stores and releases it. Because of this, Liver Chi is important for the vitality of all parts of the body.

Weakness in the Liver can be seen in the eyes and tendons. Aching knees are one indicator of weakness; jaundiced eyes are another. When the Liver Chi is weak, we may suffer from too much anger or irritation or be unable to express anger at all.[28] Anger management problems can lead to Liver problems. But when the Liver is healthy, we find kindness easy to offer; by offering kindness we can help to heal our liver.

The Fu Organs

The fu Organs are the receptor Organs. These hollow, yang-like Organs receive the fluids and energies from their zang counterparts. They excrete wastes and receive, digest, absorb, and transmit nutrients. We can generalize and say that the fu Organs transform and transmit.

The Small Intestines

Paired with the Heart, the Small Intestines receive and store water and food. Just as we understand in the West, the Small Intestines are believed to digest food, convert it into nutrition, and send the unusable bits downward for excretion. A Chinese doctor would call the bits for excretion "turbid" and the nutritious bits "clear." If we are suffering from too much heat or too much dampness, problems may arise in our urinary system and turbidity will increase.

The Stomach

Paired with the Spleen, the Stomach receives and digests food. It also stores food and water. If Stomach Chi is weak, food stagnates and all manner of digestive problems arise.

The Large Intestine

Paired with the Lungs, the Large Intestines compact our solid wastes. Just as the Lungs' Chi controls water, the Large Intestines also affect water through the ability to absorb it. Too little absorption and we suffer loose bowels, too much and we become constipated.

The Urinary Bladder

Paired with the Kidneys, the Urinary Bladder stores and excretes urine. If there are problems with Kidney Chi, this may show up in problems such as frequent urination or the need to get up at night many times to urinate.

The Gall Bladder

Paired with the Liver, the Gall Bladder stores and excretes bile. (In Chinese medicine, bile is considered to be Liver Chi, not the byproduct of the liver's digestion of fats, as we believe in the West.) Together with the Liver, the Gall Bladder builds and controls the blood and our overall Chi levels. When weak, the Gall Bladder may cause us to be indecisive or hesitant. When strong, the Gall Bladder allows us to be decisive and bold.

The San Jiao

This Organ has no Western counterpart. Sometimes referred to as the Triple Burner, this Organ's function relates to digestion and overall elimination. There are many views of what the San Jiao is and does, but it is often considered to have three separable functions and locations: [29]

▷ The Upper Jiao, located above the diaphragm, distributes water in a mist form throughout the body, assisting the Heart and Lungs;

▷ The Middle Jiao, located between the diaphragm and the navel, assists the Stomach and Spleen with digestion and the transportation of nutrients;

▷ The Lower Jiao, located below the navel, assists the Kidneys and Urinary Bladder in their roles of elimination.

Beyond the zang and fu Organs listed here, there are six other miscellaneous Organs in the Chinese models. These organs of consciousness are associated with Jing energy and include the Brain, Bone Marrow, Blood Vessels, Uterus, Gall Bladder (again!), and the Meridians, which are described below.

The Meridians

Meridian is the English translation of the Chinese word for the channels that conduct energy throughout the body. These conduits form a network. If the network is disrupted, if blockages occur, the body will not function properly: if Chi, Jing, and Shen do not flow as required, the Organs will not perform their function, and imbalance arises. When the meridians are clear and open, energy flows freely and all is well.

When we looked at the highways within our subtle body from the yogic perspective, we discovered the ancient yogis sensed thousands upon thousands of individual passageways, which they called the nadis. Both Indian and Daoist maps show that our bodies are full of conduits for the subtle energies that flow within us. [30]

As in India, the Chinese psychonauts realized that not all channels are equally important. In China, with a greater concern over physical well-being and longevity, seventy-one meridians were named and of these, fourteen were most important. Each of the ten major Organs has its associated meridian, and the meridian may be yin or yang, depending upon the zang or fu nature of the Organ. The pericardium and San Jiao also have their associated meridians, which, along with the others, make up twelve major meridians known as *Jing Mai*. We will later discover two additional significant channels that bring the total number of major meridians to fourteen.

We will limit our investigation to these major meridians. There are six that begin or end in the feet. Relative to their position in the body these can be considered yin meridians, compared to another six that begin or end in the hands, which can be considered yang meridians. As yin meridians, these lower ones are more strongly affected during a Yin Yoga practice than the higher yang meridians. We will begin our investigation with these six lower lines.[31] We will describe each meridian as a single line, but usually there are two meridians— one for each side of the body.

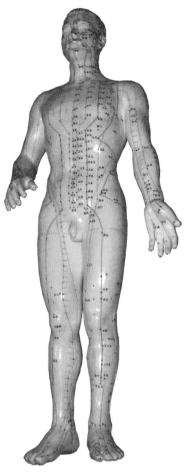

Mr. Meridian Man

The Lower Body Meridians

These six meridians are the lines affected most by the yin asanas. This certainly does not mean we cannot stress the other meridian lines during our Yin Yoga work; we can and do, but since Yin Yoga primarily affects the region from the navel to the knees, these lower six are targeted more frequently.

The Liver Meridian

The Liver meridian begins at the inside of the nail of the big toe and runs along the top of the foot. It climbs the front of the ankle and then runs up the inside of the leg until it reaches the pubic area. From here it curves around the external genitalia and goes into the lower abdomen[32] where it enters the liver and gall bladder. Rising higher, it branches in several directions, with one branch connecting to the Lung meridian. Rising still higher, it follows the throat and connects with the eyes before branching again. One branch reaches down across the cheeks and circles the lips, while a higher one crosses the forehead to the crown, where it links with the Governor Vessel meridian.

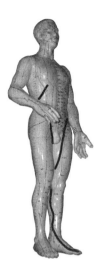

Lower back pain, abdominal pain, or mental disturbances may be a sign of disharmony of the Liver. Frequent or unreasonable anger or irritation may also be a sign of dysfunction here.

The Gall Bladder Meridian

The Gall Bladder meridian begins at the outer corner of the eye and immediately branches into two lines. A main branch remains on the surface and winds back and forth across the side of the head and above the ear, before turning downward along the side of the neck. After following the top of the shoulder, it passes under the arm and zigzags along the side of the ribs to the hips. The other branch goes inside the cheek and descends to the liver and gall bladder. From there it descends farther and rejoins the first branch at the front of the hip. The single line then descends, running along the outside thigh and knee until it reaches the ankle. It runs across the top of the foot until it reaches the fourth toe; another branch leaves at the ankle to run across the top of the foot and join the Liver meridian at the big toe.

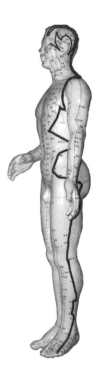

Headache, blurred vision, and pains along the side of the body including the eyes, ears, and throat may be an indication of problems with the Gall Bladder meridian.

The Kidney Meridian

The Kidney meridian begins at the outside of the little toe and immediately goes under the sole of the foot. It follows the arch, makes a circle around the inner ankle, runs through the heel, comes up the inmost side of the leg,

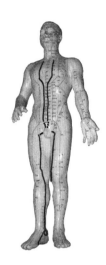

and into the tailbone. It follows the spine to the kidney and then branches. One branch heads to the urinary bladder, where it comes back to the surface of the abdomen and up the chest, ending at the clavicle. The other branch touches the liver and diaphragm and moves up through the lungs and throat until it ends beside the root of the tongue.

Disharmony here is suggested by gynecological problems, genital disorders, and problems in the kidneys, lungs, and throat. Examples may include impotence, frequent urination, and weakness in the lower limbs. Anxiety and fear may also occur.

The Urinary Bladder Meridian

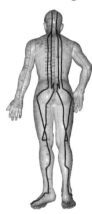

The Urinary Bladder meridian starts at the inner eye and then goes up, across the forehead, and to the crown. One branch splits here, enters the brain, and then reemerges at the scapula and runs just inside the line of the scapula down the spine to the buttocks, where it reenters the body and runs to the urinary bladder and the kidney. The second branch from the crown flows down the back of the neck and shoulder and runs just outside and parallel to the first branch. This branch continues down the back of the buttocks and legs, circles the outer ankle, runs along the outer edge of the foot, and ends in the small toe.

Signs of disharmony in the Urinary Bladder may include backaches, headaches, an inability to urinate, mental problems, and disease of the lower limbs.

The Spleen Meridian

Starting at the inside of the big toe, the Spleen meridian runs along the inside of the foot, then turns and runs up the inside of the ankle and the shin. Up to the knee, it runs just above the Liver meridian, then it runs along the top of the thigh and enters the abdominal cavity, just above the pubic bone.

It connects to the spleen and then the stomach, where it branches. The main branch comes to the surface and runs up the chest to the throat, where it again enters the body, going to the root of the tongue, where it spreads out. The second branch remains internal and reaches the heart, connecting to the Heart meridian.

Indications of Spleen disharmony include stomach problems, flatulence, vomiting, and bloating. Unreasonable worry may also arise.

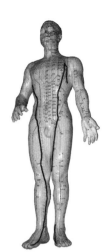

The Stomach Meridian

Beginning at the side of the nose, the Stomach meridian rises to the corner of the eye before descending along the side of the nose. Entering the upper gum, it follows the outer lips to the lower jaw, toward the joint of the jaw. Here, one branch ascends along the front of the ear to the forehead. The other branch descends through the body to the diaphragm and runs to the stomach and spleen. A third branch emerges from the lower jaw and runs across the outside of the body, crossing the chest and belly, until it terminates in the groin. The line that runs through the stomach reconnects with this third branch and runs downward along the front of the leg, reaching the top of the foot. Here it splits again, with the main branch ending in the outside tip of the second toe. The other branch reaches the inner side of the big toe. Just below the knee an additional branch splits off and runs to the lateral side of the third toe.

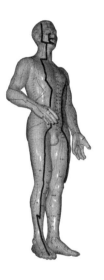

Problems with the Stomach meridian may be indicated by bloating, vomiting, pain in any of the areas the meridian passes through (mouth, nose, teeth, etc.), and mental problems.

The Upper Body Meridians

There are six meridians that begin or end in the fingers. They all pass through the shoulder or armpit. While our normal Yin Yoga practice does not target these lines specifically, it is possible to affect all our meridians during a Yin Yoga practice.[33]

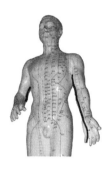

The Heart Meridian

The three branches of the Heart meridian begin in the heart. One branch flows downward through the diaphragm to meet the small intestines. Another rises up alongside the throat and ends in the eye. The third runs across the chest, through the lungs, and comes out through the armpit. It flows along the midline of the inside upper arm, through the inner elbow, along the midline of the inner lower arm, until it crosses the wrist and palm and ends in the inside tip of the little finger, where it connects to the Small Intestine meridian.

Disorders of the heart and chest such as palpitations, pain, insomnia, night sweats, and mental problems may signal problems with this meridian.

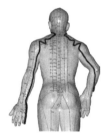

The Small Intestine Meridian

The Small Intestine meridian begins at the outer tip of the little finger. It runs along the back edge of the hand, through the wrist, upward along the outer forearm and upper arm, to the shoulder. After circling the back of the shoulder, it meets the Governor Vessel meridian. Here it branches, with one branch going inside the body and descending through the heart, diaphragm, and stomach before ending in the small intestine. Another branch ascends along the side of the neck to the cheek and outer corner of the eye and then goes to the ear. Another small branch leaves the cheek to run to the inner eye, where it meets the Urinary Bladder meridian.

Disharmony may be indicated by ear, eye, or stomach problems such as deafness, pain in the lower abdomen, or pain in the shoulders or neck.

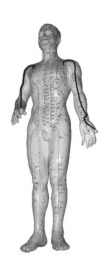

The Lung Meridian

The Lung meridian begins inside the belly just above the navel and drops down to the large intestines. From here it comes back up through the diaphragm and connects to the stomach. It ascends through the lungs and follows the throat before coming to the front of the shoulder from under the clavicle. From here it runs along the outer, thumb side of the upper arm and the front of the lower arm. It crosses the wrist and ends at the outer tip of the thumb. A small branch goes from the wrist to the tip of the index finger, where it connects to the Large Intestine meridian.

Respiratory problems like coughs, asthma, and chest pains may signify dysfunction. Extreme and persistent sadness and grief may also indicate problems here.

The Large Intestine Meridian

Beginning at the tip of the index finger, the Large Intestine meridian runs between the thumb and forefinger and along the outside of the arm. It comes over the outside top of the shoulder and along the back of the shoulder blades to the spine. Here, one branch descends through the lungs, diaphragm, and large intestines. The second branch ascends along the neck and lower cheek and enters the lower gum, circling the lower teeth. On the outside, this line also circles the upper lips, crosses under the nose, and rises up to join the Stomach meridian.

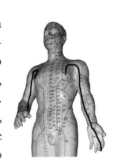

Problems in the mouth, teeth, nose, and throat such as toothaches and sore throats, as well as problems with the neck and shoulders, may indicate disharmony.

The Pericardium Meridian

The pericardium covers the heart and is considered in Chinese medicine to be an Organ of its own. The Pericardium meridian begins in the chest and connects to the pericardium. From here it moves down the chest, connecting the three sections of the San Jiao meridian. Another branch moves horizontally across the chest, coming to the surface of the ribs, up and around the armpit, and down the front of the bicep and forearm to the palm, ending at the tip of the middle finger. A small branch leads from the palm to the tip of the ring finger, where it connects to the San Jiao meridian.

Pain in the heart area, poor circulation, stomach problems, and mental problems may indicate disharmony of the Pericardium meridian.

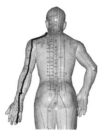

The San Jiao Meridian

The San Jiao meridian is often called the Triple Burner or Triple Energizer. It begins in the ring finger, where the Pericardium meridian ends. It runs over the back of the hand, wrist, and lower arm. It passes the outer point of the elbow and the back of the upper arm to the posterior shoulder. From here it comes over the shoulder to the front of the body and enters the chest beneath the sternum. It branches, with the main branch running to the pericardium and continuing down through the diaphragm to the three burners: upper, middle, and lower. The second branch ascends along the side of the neck, circles the back of the ear, and then circles the side of the face. Another small branch emerges from the back of the ear and connects to the Gall Bladder meridian at the outer corner of the eye.

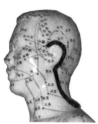

Problems associated with this meridian may occur in the side of the face, neck, or throat, or in the abdomen. Examples include deafness, ringing in the ears, bloating, and urinary difficulties.

The Extra Meridians

The meridian system is made up of the lines connecting the five yin and six yang organs, plus the pericardium. Beyond these twelve, there are eight additional meridians that a Chinese doctor must know. We will visit the two most important: the Governor Vessel and the Conception Vessel meridians. These are important because they have acupuncture points separate from those on any of the other twelve main meridians. All the other extra meridians share points with the main meridians.

The Governor Vessel

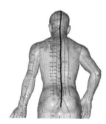

The Governor Vessel begins within the lower belly and splits in three. Two smaller branches ascend to connect to each kidney. The third and main branch descends to the perineum, where it enters the tip of the spinal cord and rises up to the brain. This branch comes over the top of the skull, down the middle of the forehead and nose, and terminates in the upper gum. Dr. Motoyama recommends the practice of Nadi Shodhana to purify this meridian.[34]

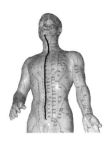

The Conception Vessel

This meridian also begins in the lower abdomen next to the Governor Vessel. It has only one branch and it, too, descends to the perineum. Emerging from the muladhara, it ascends along the front midline of the body through the neck and chin to the mouth. At the mouth it splits and goes around the lips before sending branches to the lower eyes.

The Governor Vessel and Conception Vessel run along the front and back of the torso. These lines also contain the front and back of each chakra. When we breathe and draw energy up the Governor Vessel and down the Conception Vessel, we are completing the microcosmic orbit.

Acupuncture and Acupressure

The meridian lines that we just looked at flow along the surface of the body and deep inside as well. The interior lines are more important than those on the outside, but along the exterior paths there are special locations, known as acupuncture points, where stimulation will increase or enhance the flow of the various textures through the meridians. There are two ways we can stimulate these points, acupuncture and acupressure.

The practice of acupuncture goes back over 2,000 years. While many high cultures utilized massage, breath work, exercises, special herbs and other dietary prescriptions to enhance health and longevity, the Daoists are unique in their use of needles. The earliest needles were probably bone or bamboo, but it didn't take long for metal needles to come into vogue, with silver and gold being the favorites. In modern times, disposable stainless steel needles are used.

How deeply the needles are inserted depends upon where they are being used: a few millimeters may be enough in the hands, but two or three inches may be required in the buttocks. Often a dozen or more will be required in any one session. Sometimes the needles are just left in, quietly, and other times they are jiggled or heated. Generally a dull, achy sensation is felt: this shows that the needles are in fact doing something. What they are doing is rebalancing the energies: what is stagnant will circulate; what is deficient will increase; what is cold will be warmed. Chi and Blood will be affected and thus all the textures of the body will be affected. Each meridian line upon which the acupuncture points lie pertains to a specific Organ pair, so these Organs will also benefit from the procedure.

There are other ways to stimulate the flows of energy, as we saw in the section on moving energy in chapter 2. In our Yin Yoga practice we stimulate the flow of Chi through acupressure. While not as precise as acupuncture, by simply massaging, compressing or stretching the tissues that lie along the meridian lines we can also stimulate energy flow and rebalance our systems. For example, if we feel a strong tugging along the inner groins while in Straddle pose, we are stimulating the Liver and Kidney meridians. If we feel a tugging along the outside of the hips in full Swan and compression along the lower back due to the backbend, we are stimulating the Gall Bladder and Urinary Bladder meridians.

In general, every time we come into a Yin Yoga pose, we should pay attention to where we are feeling the stress. Check the pictures shown earlier to see which meridian lines run along the areas where the stress is significant and you will discover which meridian lines you are stimulating. You will find that we often are stimulating several lines at once. Remember too that the meridian lines will feed more than one Organ: stimulating the Gall Bladder in Swan also benefits the Liver. And, any time we stimulate the Kidneys, because they are the home of Jing, we benefit all other Organs.

If you are feeling it, you are doing it! Now, just notice where you are feeling it.

Emotions

Sometimes what we are feeling is not just physical sensations in the body, but strong emotions. The Daoist yogis noticed that our emotions are embodied. Modern yogis have noticed the same thing and coined the term "issues in our tissues." Our Organs are the home of emotions: the Heart contains both love and exuberance; our Liver contains kindness and anger. Our Kidneys can be the source of fear or the source of deep-seated wisdom. Each Organ not only houses certain emotions but our emotions can affect the pertaining Organs. Too much fear can deplete Kidney energy (Jing). Conversely, if we have too little Jing we may become fearful.

The Indian yogis noticed a correlation between our bodies and our heart. Don't be surprised if, during a deep Yin Yoga practice, emotions start to surface. This is part of the practice. Just as we can have physical scar tissues that need to be broken through, we may also have emotional scar tissue to work through. Hip openers will often elicit feelings of frustration, annoyance, and anger. Hips openers tend to massage the Gall Bladder meridian and its partner, the Liver, which is the home of anger and frustration.

Deep backbends may create feelings of fear or anxiety: here we are working deeply into the Kidneys, which are the home of fear and wisdom. If you can acknowledge your fear, wisdom will grow. If you can be with your anger, kindness may blossom.

If you are going through a very emotional time, you may wish to structure your yoga practice to work the meridian lines that support the Organ housing that emotion. Grief and sadness, which reside in the Lungs, may be helped by working the Lung meridians through working the upper body, specifically the arms and shoulders. Worry may be moderated by working the Stomach and Spleen meridians through deep stretches of the thighs and front side of the torso.

Remember to play your edges: don't push too far, too fast. If you are not ready for an emotional release, don't force it. Wait for the heart to open over time. If the emotional sensations are manageable, then let them marinate. We don't have to react to the emotions that arise during our practice; we just need to notice them. Acknowledge what you are feeling and be curious. Yin is allowing: allow what is surfacing to be there, without running away from it or trying to change it—if that is the appropriate response.

If we heal the body we also heal the heart. Emotional imbalances can be addressed through our practice, which in turn may cure some physiological imbalances. The Daoist maps explain how this happens: our emotions are rooted in the organs and our organs affect our emotions. What we do to one, we do to the other. Yin Yoga works the total person: our body, heart, mind, and soul.

A Western View

In India, the yogic sages observed ten forms of prana through subjective experience. In China, the Daoists mapped thirty-two forms of Chi. Some seers have intuited even more than this number. To our Western ways of thinking, these subjective claims seem fanciful and unsubstantiated by objective study. When asked, most Westerns will say that our bodies use two kinds of energy: chemical and electrical. That's it! But is that really all there is?

Chemical energy is transmitted via the blood system. Electrical energy is transmitted via the nervous system. These are the two great communication systems we are aware of, but consider a primitive amoeba: it has no internal vascular system but if it is injured it will repair itself. A primitive animal, like a sponge, will repair itself even though it has no central nervous system. Obviously, long before there were blood systems and nervous systems, communication and healing were possible within an organism. There is more going on within our bodies than are mapped in our Western models. Fortunately, many researchers are hard at work extending our maps to include energy features that the yogis in the East may have been describing.

In this section we will review just some of the new findings in a field called Energy Medicine. We will begin with a brief primer on electricity and magnetism.

New Paradigms

Wholeness—health—requires communication internally and the ability to move substances. The cells of the body need to communicate with each other. When this communication breaks down we cannot remain whole. The same point applies to transporting energy and materials within the body. Consider the example of a city during a blackout. When the power is down, transportation is shut down, communication ceases, and the city stops functioning. The body is similar; we need information and energy to flow, whether this is chemical information in the form of substances moving from one area of the body to another or electrical information informing one area of what is happening in another area. Ill health can be considered, in this model, as a failure in the communication and transportation network of the body.

For more than five hundred million years complex life has been evolving and finding ways to improve the ability to communicate and transport energy and information within a body. Through trial and error life has found ways to do this better and better—which means faster, more accurately, and with backup systems in case of problems. Nature and her laws of physics provide many possible methods to choose from. The most successful forms of life would naturally adopt as many of these as possible.

The earliest multicellular life forms used chemical means to communicate. Materials were physically passed from one cell to the next. Then conduits were created within which these substances could travel farther, faster, and more surely. These conduits evolved into our blood system. The nervous system evolved in a similar manner.

A new paradigm is evolving in the West, one that broadens the scope of information and energy transportation mechanisms far beyond simple chemical and electrical models. This new paradigm includes many other forms of communication and energy movement, which were hinted at by doctors in centuries past.[35] With our modern, sensitive instruments, capable of detecting minute levels of energy, we are able to test these new models. We are going to explore just a couple of these new models, starting with bioelectricity—the electricity of the body.

Bioelectricity

Have you noticed the shoes worn by children that light up as they run? Kids love the flashing light show put on by their shoes and parents love the fact that no batteries are needed. Where does the electricity come from to spark the lights? The answer is piezoelectricity—electricity created by pressure. The word comes from the Greek *piezein,* which means to squeeze or compress. No batteries required.[36]

Certain kinds of crystals, when subjected to deforming stress, create electrical fields or cause electricity to flow. The reverse can also happen: when an electric field is applied to these crystals they will bend in response—the stronger the field the greater the deformation; the greater the stress the stronger the field.

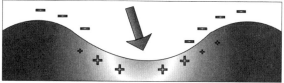

Piezoelectric crystals do not need to be recharged. When they resume their original shape the energy potential ends, and when they are deformed again the field is regenerated. This wonderful ability of some crystals has been exploited in many technologies today. From the light show in shoes to barbecues' ignition, electric microphones, and sophisticated sonar systems—piezoelectricity has become commonplace.

A crystal is a structured array of molecules repeated throughout the material. What is often overlooked is that tissues in our body are also aligned in structured, repeating patterns. The molecules of our muscles, bones, eyes, cell membranes, collagen, elastin, even our DNA—all have crystal-like structure.

James Oschman, in his excellent books summarizing scientific research and energy medicine, states that the living tissues of our bodies are best described as liquid crystals, materials that are intermediate between solids and liquids and display properties of both.[37] He explains that virtually the whole body is composed of materials arranged in a liquid crystal form and cites several studies confirming this model.

When our liquid crystalline tissues are subjected to deforming stress, they generate piezoelectric potential energy and tiny electric currents. Just like in the children's shoes, every move we make, every breath we take (to paraphrase Sting), creates tiny currents of energy.

If these piezoelectric energies we are discussing were expected to move materials in our body or affect us in large ways, we would be right to think they have no chance of affecting us. But consider this metaphor: You are cooking a big Thanksgiving turkey (or, for vegetarian yogis, a Tofurky™). You need to preheat the oven, but you don't know how high to set it. You call your mother on your cell phone, and she tells you to try 400 degrees Fahrenheit. The cell phone consumes a very small amount of electricity, say 50 milliwatts. The oven produces a great deal of heat and requires 1,000 watts to run properly.[38] And yet, until the small current in the cell phone gives you the information you need, all that power in the oven is dormant. Certainly the cell phone could not hope to power the oven. But without the cell phone's intelligence, the power in the oven would never be activated. A small amount of information can create big changes. And this small amount of information requires very little power compared to the large effect it stimulates.

If our bodies can be considered as liquid crystals, and if even small movements create electric fields and currents, this could provide a basis for scientific models of information and energy transfers beyond purely chemical or electrical mechanisms, which solely rely on our nervous system or blood system. With such models we can begin to see how modalities that manipulate the body physically, such as yoga and massage, might have an effect on the functioning of our bodies and our health.

Bioelectricity and Our Bones

We have already seen that Yin Yoga can fight degeneration of our bones. One of the many tissues that are structured in a crystalline array is our bone tissue. When we stress our bones, we create little piezoelectric currents within the bone itself. This current signals the cells within the bones and affects their behaviors. There are cells in our bones whose job it is to create new bone, called osteoblasts, and there are cells whose job it is to clean up old, worn-out bones, called osteoclasts. If we actively stress our bones, through yoga, walking, or other weight-bearing exercises, we are telling our osteoclasts to slow down their destruction of older bone, which allows the osteoblasts to continue to build new bone, thus making our bones thicker and stronger. Without stress on the bones, they become hollowed out by the continuous action of the osteoclasts. We need to stress the bones so that we create electrical currents that slow down degeneration.

This is not just happening within our bones: these piezoelectric currents are occurring all over our body, guiding our cells to either get busy or slow down. Another form of electrical signaling, again occurring outside our central nervous system, is the injury repair current. This is a small current that is created in our tissues when they are damaged, and it is used to signal to various cells that help is needed. This current does not flow through our nervous system but it is able to attract immune cells, fibroblasts and other cells needed to repair the damage. When the repairs are completed, the current ceases.

Electromagnetism

There are two basic kinds of magnets: permanent magnets and electromagnets. The permanent magnets are familiar to everyone; they're what attach notes to the door of your fridge. Electromagnets have a magnetic field only when an electric current is present. When we pass a current through a wire, a magnetic field is created all around the wire. If we reverse the direction of the current, the orientation of the magnetic field also reverses.

A moving electron creates both electric and magnetic fields. It is therefore better to consider electric and magnetic fields as aspects of a more general type of field, known as the electromagnetic field. When we use this term we are referring to either or both of the electrical field and/or the magnetic field.

There are naturally occurring electromagnetic fields and artificially created ones. The earth has a very large magnetic field compared to the fields inside our bodies. The earth's field arises from many sources including lightning, which creates electromagnetic fields even stronger than the earth's but last only for a very short time. The electrical wires outside and inside your home all have their own electromagnetic fields. They also arise from your fridge magnets and stereo speakers. These household fields are far stronger than the earth's magnetic field, but are not as pervasive.

Our hearts have an electric current regulating them, as well as an electromagnetic field. The size of our heart's magnetic field is one million times smaller than the earth's magnetic field and it, too, can vary from person to person and from time to time within the same person. Despite its weakness, the electromagnetic field of the heart is measurable. Electrocardiograms (ECGs) are used to measure the electrical force at various locations throughout the body.[39] Our brains are also a source of electrical activity and have a measurable field. The brain's magnetic field is around a thousand times weaker than the heart's and naturally was not detected until long after the heart's field was discovered.

Any electrons that are in motion will give rise to an electromagnetic field. What about those tiny piezoelectric fields discussed in the previous section? Do they create electromagnetic fields and, if so, can they be measured? These tiny fields, while too small to have been detected until recently, do exist and their associated electromagnetic fields have been measured, thanks to the invention of a cool-sounding device known as a SQUID.[40] Invented by John Zimmerman in the early 1970s, a SQUID allows magnetometers to detect very small electromagnetic fields. Zimmerman, and others after him, were able to detect an increase in the electromagnetic field of a therapeutic touch from a practitioner's hands.[41] The study of these generated electromagnetic fields is called bioelectromagnetism.

Bioelectromagnetism

Our blood is mostly water with a lot of salts and minerals dissolved within it. Water saturated like this turns out to be an excellent conductor for electricity. It is not surprising that an ECG will pick up signals from the heart throughout the body: the field is propagated via the blood system. The heart's electrical field touches every part of us, and its magnetic field is also pervasive. The signals from the heart have been speculated to send information throughout our matrix. The heart is not just a pump: it is the center of a communication system that can let the whole body know what is happening.

Unfortunately, in earlier standard medical paradigms the presence of the body's electric fields was useful only as a diagnostic tool; these models could not predict any therapeutic procedures that could utilize the electric or magnetic fields of the body. As we will see, alternative medicine practitioners have used this knowledge in a therapeutic way.

So far we have discussed only how an electron in motion gives rise to a magnetic field. The reverse is also true. A moving magnetic field can create an electrical current. This is how an electric generator works: a magnet is placed within a coil of wires. When the magnet is rotated, electricity is created. Conversely, if electricity is run through the coil, the magnet rotates; that is the basis for an electric motor. Not only do our bodies create magnetic fields, they can also be affected by them.

After inventing the SQUID, John Zimmerman began some interesting research on the magnetic fields of touch therapists. A similar but more detailed study was done later in Japan.[42] The Japanese study included not just therapists but also Chi-gong masters, Zen masters, yogis, and meditators. The results of these studies showed that a therapeutic touch specialist emitted from her hands magnetic fields that were 100 to 1,000 times stronger than our heart's field. The studies also revealed that the magnetic fields were pulsating at low frequencies, ranging from 0.3–30 Hz.[43] Most of the magnetic field frequencies centered around 7–8 Hz but the fields continuously spanned the range of frequencies. Of course, the therapists had no idea of what they were doing; they were just doing their thing.[44]

Bioelectromagnetic Healing

All of this is fascinating, but why is it important? Since the early 1800s, scientists and doctors have experimented with magnets for their possible therapeutic benefits. In the late 1800s, when medicine became standardized, this research was stopped. Recently, however, it has begun again. The findings of these more modern researchers have vindicated the earlier beliefs that magnetism can help people heal in certain situations. One therapy is called pulsed electromagnetic field (PEMF) therapy.

Here's how it works: Occasionally, when someone suffers a broken bone, the bone doesn't heal. The doctor sets the bone, perhaps applies a cast, but after several months, the bone is still fractured. After several years, it is still broken! This is known as a non-union fracture. Somehow something has gone wrong with the repair mechanism in the body. The information needed to heal the fracture is not getting to the tissues responsible for fixing the break. Today, many doctors know that PEMF will help. A magnetic field generator is placed around the broken bone and an oscillating magnetic field is applied for eight to ten hours every day. Clinical tests have shown that even for broken bones that have remained unhealed for forty years, they can be repaired with this technique.[45]

The frequency of the magnetic field applied to a broken bone is 7 Hz. This healing frequency is called the "frequency window of specificity" (FWS). Sisken and Walker in 1995 reported that various FWS affect different issues.

FREQUENCY	EFFECTS
2 Hz	Nerve regeneration
7 Hz	Bone growth
10 Hz	Ligament repair
15–20 Hz	Skin repair
25 and 50 Hz	Assistance with nerve growth

While Zimmerman's investigations of the magnetic fields emitted by touch therapists did not prove that healing was occurring, he did discover that the therapists were emitting magnetic fields that spanned the same frequencies that other scientists discovered stimulated healing. Future studies are required to prove that healing touch can actually heal, but these results have pointed to a promising area of investigation.

Let's reflect for a moment what this means to us as we do our yoga practice. All yoga practices stress our tissues, and this pressure creates piezoelectric currents. These currents send information through our tissues and communicate what is happening so that proper cellular responses can occur. These currents also create magnetic fields, which can also trigger healing responses. As we stretch, twist, and compress our muscles and connective tissues we are energetically turning ourselves on, literally.

Energy Pathways

When required information is not provided to an injured or sick area of the body, the body's own resources are not mobilized to respond or the body responds ineffectually or even inappropriately. Alternative healing modalities such as yoga, Tai Chi, massage, energy manipulation therapies, and many others could be ways of injecting the missing information through very weak, low-frequency electromagnetic field generation. Let's complete the construction of a possible model by looking more closely, at the cellular level, at how this information may be transmitted.

Electrical fields follow the flow of electricity. As we have seen, the nerves are not the only conductors of electricity in the body. An ECG measures the electrical activity of the heart in places far away from our chest. These signals are possible because the blood system itself conducts electromagnetic information. So the circulatory system is one possible channel for electromagnetic energy, not just chemical energy. Interestingly, the Daoists long ago identified the Blood system as a conduit of Chi. If Chi is not simply chemical energy perhaps they were sensing this conductance of electromagnetic energy through our blood vessels. Or, perhaps, the definition of Chi needs to be broadened to include all these forms of energy: chemical, electrical, and electromagnetic.

Does it stop there? Does our circulatory system feed every part of the body? What about inside the cells? How can information be transmitted to the insides of the cells themselves? To answer this question we need to look at the current and the evolving models of the cell.

The Bag of Soup Model

In most books that describe the anatomy of a cell, you will find lovely diagrams showing all the organelles, the major components of a cell, floating in a pool of liquid. These models are very elegant and detailed, but what is that water-like substance inside the cell? Soup! In an early popular model of the cell, all the internal apparatus float in this soup. Materials from outside the cell ease their way past the permeable cell membrane and then drift around in the soup until they happen to bump into something important. The chemical energy model of communication requires a random movement of these chemicals until they find and latch onto their destination.

This is not a very satisfying model, relying as it does on random timing for information transfers to occur. James Oschman notes that many cellular activities happen much faster than a random walkabout would allow. Something is missing in this model.[46]

When we look in most anatomy books and see the way the body is depicted, we find a similar "something missing." The pictures will show in wonderful detail the circulatory system, or they may trace the skeletal system or the muscular or nervous systems. But all these models omit the material that these systems are embedded within. What is missing is the connective tissue. Connective tissues join the circulatory system to the nervous system to the muscular system and so on. Our connective tissues are ubiquitous and, as we have seen, are formed of collagen fibers, elastin fibers, and many other components arrayed in crystalline matrices. These matrices form the piezoelectric crystals that create and conduct the electrical energies we were discussing in the previous section.

These matrices are exactly what are missing in the bag of soup cellular models. We need a new model that fills in the gaps and explains the cellular processes more completely.

The Cytoskeleton

Newer models of the cell's anatomy recognize that the cell is not just a bag of goo. There is a structure inside it. As illustrated below, the cell is filled with fibers and filaments, tubes and structure. Collectively this structure is called the cytoskeleton or the cytoplasmic matrix and, just like our body's bony skeleton, it provides rigidity and support to the whole cell. More than that, the cytoskeleton provides pathways for information to flow along. No longer do we have to imagine chemical information just floating around in the sea

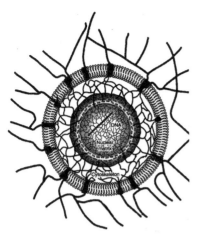

of soup waiting for a chance encounter. Now we find that chemical information can be guided to its destination by enzymes that line the cytoskeleton.

Notice that the lines forming the cytoskeleton extend out beyond the cell walls. These linking elements are called integrins, and they connect the inner and outer worlds of our cells. We have already seen that the extra-cellular matrix is networked via our fascia throughout our whole body. With each cell connected inside and outside, with the ground substance flowing everywhere throughout the body, we find that every cell has a connection to every other cell in our body. There is no place that is not connected to every other place within us.

We have said this complete interconnection is potentially so. We have also postulated that illness is a blocking of information, an inability of the body to transmit healing signals to the affected area. If a problem isolates one region of the body from the others, information may not get through. Like a city suffering a power outage, communication lines may be out of service, transportation systems may fail. The city may survive for a short time but unless outside help arrives, the city is doomed. Our body is not very different. Health means wholeness. If one part of the body is cut off from the information flow throughout the body, illness arises.

Meridians Revisited

Western scientists who originally investigated the Eastern claims of meridians and nadis went back to their dissection tables looking for physical manifestations of these channels. Their dissections discarded the supposedly inert connective tissues. They looked past these tissues searching for something that just wasn't there. They looked for channels and conducting tubes similar to nerves and blood vessels, and could not find them. Their conclusion: no channels, no meridians. Ironically, they discarded the very tissues that formed the channels they were seeking. Energies flow through the connective tissues, through the water-hugging fibers of the ground substance.

The ancient sages told us that there were 72,000 nadis. Some said 300,000: some said 350,000. They were wrong: the number of connections between the trillions of cells in our body is beyond counting.[47] Are these connections the nadis and the meridians that the sages explored? Are they the conduits of the energies of prana and Chi? Are these energies and channels what the early psychonauts were trying to map with the cultural concepts they had at their disposal?

What about the thirty-two different forms of Chi that the Daoists detected? In his studies, Dr. Oschman also investigated gravitational information, infrared, photonic, microwave, and many other forms of energy that the body seems to employ to communicate information. It does indeed seem likely that, over hundreds of millions of years of evolution, life on earth has adapted to, and adopted, everything Mother Nature has made available to us. When we add these forms of energies to the ones we have already talked about (chemical, electrical, and magnetic) and the myriad of ways that we are discovering that cells signal each other, the total exceeds the number the sages gave us. Once again, rather than finding that the Indian and Daoist yogis were exaggerating, we can speculate that they were being rather conservative in their descriptions of what is going on inside our bodies.

Acupuncture Revisited

In 1997 the National Institutes of Health (NIH) removed the "experimental" label from the use of acupuncture and noted that acupuncture can be effective at reducing post-chemotherapy and nausea during pregnancy, and shows some pain relief for certain conditions. The NIH conducted a multi-year study into the many claims of acupuncture benefits, but while there were some scientific studies done with proper controls, most studies lacked controls and were inadequate. While acupuncture was found to be efficacious for pain and nausea, conventional Western medical treatments such as analgesics also dealt with these conditions without having to subject patients to the pain and trouble of being "needled."[48]

By 2009 several rigorous studies had been conducted that showed acupuncture can indeed change the brain's perception of pain, and there are some indications that acupuncture can help with other conditions such as irritable bowel syndrome and depression.[49] Another study showed that acupuncture can be effective even without the needles![50] All we need to do is stress the acupuncture point, which of course is acupressure. In some cases it was found that a simple pinch was all that was needed to stimulate endorphin releases in the brain.[51]

Clearly the Western point of view about acupuncture is still evolving. It is doubtful that all the extravagant claims of the vast array of benefits from acupuncture will remain when more study is done, but it is also quite clear that something is happening when we stimulate these acupuncture points and meridians, whether with or without needles. What could this "something" be?

There is, again, no consensus on how acupuncture works, and there may indeed be several mechanisms involved. One speculation is that acupuncture needling simulates an injury, which causes an injury-repair current to be generated. If this current is generated in a place where there is a communication channel, perhaps some low-resistance pathway through the water-filled extracellular matrix, then this current can travel through the body to some other place where it can stimulate a healing response.[52] Another speculation is that when we compress a point (acupressure), or when the acupuncture needle is jiggled or twisted, it mechanically tugs on the collagen and elastin fibers in the connective tissue. The mechanical tugging affects the nearby cells and their integrins, so in effect the stress goes right inside the cells. Reorganization of the cytoskeleton can cause cell migration, contraction and secretion of various proteins. All of these changes can create a cascade of effects within the extracellular matrix.[53]

Whether we understand the mechanism or not, our own experience is what is most important. Sometimes there is no map for where we are going, and we will just have to create our own. There is evidence of some benefits from acupuncture and acupressure acknowledged in the West. There are many more anecdotal reports of benefits from the East. When we practice Yin Yoga we should be open to, and aware of, the changes we are experiencing, both during the practice and in the days that follow.

The Nervous System

The Indian yogis were quite clear that the nadis they were mapping for us were part of the subtle body, not easily detected and obviously not our nerves. The Daoists were equally certain that the meridians they were stimulating through acupuncture were also not nerves. But, what about our nerves? If yoga is good for all our tissues, how does our nervous system benefit from the practice?

Scientists love to break things down into components. It is easier to study subsystems and from there try to work out what the whole system does. Our nervous system consists of two main subsystems: the central nervous system (CNS), which includes the brain and the spinal cord, and the peripheral nervous system, which includes the nerves that innervate our body, and which connects to the CNS. The peripheral nervous system in turn divides into the somatic nervous system, which allows conscious control over our muscles, and the autonomic nervous system (ANS), which provides involuntary control over our viscera: our organs, glands, and smooth muscles. A map of the ANS shows it consisting of three more subsystems: the enteric nervous system, which controls our digestive tract; the sympathetic nervous system (SNS), which is responsible for our fight-or-flight response; and the parasympathetic nervous system (PNS), sometimes called our rest-and-digest response. That's a lot of capital letters, and we will only talk about the last two in detail.

The Sympathetic Nervous System

"It can be argued that stress is the number one killer in the Western world today." This quote is from Dr. Timothy McCall. In his book *Yoga as Medicine*, McCall relates that stress fuels some of the biggest health problems of our day, including diabetes, depression, osteoporosis, heart attacks, strokes, and autoimmune diseases like multiple sclerosis and rheumatoid arthritis. He also says that, while there isn't a lot of evidence that stress causes cancer, it appears to increase the odds of dying from it.[54]

Stress is unavoidable in our culture and some amount of stress is actually needed for our bodies to be strong and healthy. All exercise needs to include the dual components of stress and rest. However, when we experience too much stress and not enough rest, problems arise. In physiological terms we are hyperactive in our SNS and hypoactive in our PNS.

The SNS is our basic fight-or-flight system: it is yang-like. When our ancestors were being chased by a saber-tooth tiger or attacked by the tribe in the next valley, their SNS would strongly activate and give them the energy and focus needed to flee or fight. The brain's amygdala recognizes the threat and stimulates the hypothalamus, which in turn releases hormones that activate the pituitary gland. The pituitary then releases hormones that cause our adrenal glands to release several other hormones including adrenaline, which speeds up our heart and respiration rates, and cortisol, which temporarily enhances our immune system.

THE SYMPATHETIC NERVOUS SYSTEM
▷ Dilates pupils
▷ Reduces salivary flow
▷ Accelerates heart rate
▷ Constricts arterioles
▷ Dilates bronchi
▷ Inhibits stomach secretions
▷ Relaxes urinary bladder

THE PARASYMPATHETIC NERVOUS SYSTEM
▷ Constricts pupils
▷ Stimulates tear glands
▷ Stimulates salivary glands
▷ Reduces heart rate
▷ Constricts bronchi
▷ Stimulates stomach secretion
▷ Contracts urinary bladder
▷ Stimulates sexual arousal

Stimulating the SNS diverts blood from the digestive organs to our muscles: who needs to digest now when the most important thing is to run for our lives?

Today, our bodies react in the same way to threatening signals from our environment, but there are few saber-tooth tigers around to really scare us. Our stresses are mostly caused by our way of viewing our life, not by actual external threats. The neighboring tribe may be your ex-mother-in-law or boss. Where our ancestors might have encountered a stressful situation once or twice a week, we are faced with stressful situations constantly. Simply listening to loud music, watching the news, listening to a friend complain about her life, viewing commercials, arguing with a family member, commuting to work, eating hot or spicy foods, or watching action movies can all trigger our SNS. We are in a constant state of SNS activation—we are over-stressed.

The result of chronic stress is chronically high levels of cortisol. High cortisol levels are linked to elevated fasting-blood-sugar levels, higher blood pressure and insulin resistance. We may begin "food seeking behavior" due to our stress: Dr McCall noted a study that found stressed-out children will consume more than twice as much food as their calmer fellow students.[55] While a temporary spike in cortisol can sharpen our mental focus, a continually elevated cortisol condition will lead to poor mental abilities, decreased memory and a depressed immune system. Our blood viscosity remains too thick, causing many heart problems. Bone loss, insomnia, poor wound healing, weight gain, depression, and fatigue are all consequences.

The Parasympathetic Nervous System

The PNS is more yin-like and works in a complementary direction to the SNS: it is our rest-and-digest response. Through stimulation via the nerves running to our internal organs (primarily the vagus nerve), and through the release of acetylcholine, our heart rate slows and blood pressure drops. Blood flow that was diverted away from the intestines and reproductive organs, whose function isn't essential in an emergency, returns. When we relax, our tears can flow. Our short-term memory returns, and we can think clearly. In sum, once our SNS is turned off and our PNS turned on, we rebuild and recover our health.

The key activities that turn off the fight-or-flight system and activate the rest-and-digest system are breathing and thinking. Not just any old breath, but a proper yogic breath. A slow, deep, even breath, the ocean breath, will create a relaxed nervous system, yielding a calm mind, which in turn will help the breath become slower and more even. Not just any old thinking either: our thoughts need to be calm. A positive feedback loop between the breath and our thoughts can be established that increases the effectiveness of the PNS and increases the production of a neurotransmitter known as GABA.

The Brain on Yoga

The second most common neurotransmitter in our central nervous system is called GABA.[56] GABA decreases brain activity: it helps to turn off the lights when we are no longer home. If we are stressed, all the lights are on, even if we are not home. Similar to the parasympathetic nervous system, GABA helps to reduce our stress response. People with low levels of GABA can suffer from depression and mood and anxiety disorders: drugs are often prescribed that increase GABA. Our yoga practice, when done properly, can increase our GABA levels and turn on the PNS.

Boston University Medical Center reported in August 2010 that GABA levels and mood are positively affected by yoga practice.[57] The researchers' study showed that yoga increases GABA levels in the brain and improves our mood. But, we don't need a study (and there have been several[58]) to tell us that we feel better when we do yoga. We just need to know how to tap into the practice more deeply. What is it about yoga that makes us feel so good? One factor that has been proven to make us feel good is our breath. How we breathe when we do our yoga makes all the difference. Specifically, the ocean breath described in chapter 2 is what we need to make into a habit whenever we practice yoga, yin or yang.

Professor Luciano Bernardi, of the Italian University of Pavia, reported in a 2001 study that slowing our breath rate down positively affects our heart rate variability[59] and increases baroreflex[60] sensitivity. He studied the effects of chanting the Tibetan mantra "Om Mani Padme Hum," and he discovered the benefits were identical for people who chanted "Ave Maria." In both cases, the chanting slowed the breath down to only six breaths per minute. His conclusion was, "Rhythm formulas that involve breathing at six breaths per minute induce favorable psychological and possibly physiological effects."[61]

If we can allow our breaths to be ten seconds long (six per minute), we will get the same benefits described in Bernardi's study. We can really turn off the SNS and activate the PNS. When you settle into your Yin Yoga pose, begin the ocean breath: count to four as you inhale, pause for one count, count to four as you exhale, and again pause for one count. This is a ten-second breath—proven by Bernardi's study to be great for our heart and lungs.

Summary of Energetic Benefits

No matter if the Indian, Daoist, or Western view resonates most for you, slow ocean breaths while you are holding your Yin Yoga poses will reduce stress, activate your rest-and-digest system, improve your heart and lung function, lower blood pressure, and lead to a healthier and happier life. There are many other benefits we obtain through our Yin Yoga practice, from the energetic perspective:

▷ Awaken, enhance, and balance prana.

▷ Slow the whirling thoughts of the mind.

▷ Stimulate and awaken the kundalini serpent, leading towards eventual liberation and enlightenment.

▷ Stimulate the production and flow of Chi and Jing energies.

▷ Nourish the organs through acupressure via compression of the meridian lines.

▷ Replenish the store of Jing in our Kidneys, which in turn helps all our Organs function properly.

▷ Create tiny piezoelectric currents that stimulate optimal cellular responses.

▷ Create internal pulsed magnetic fields that can restore cellular health.

▷ Turn off the sympathetic nervous system (fight-or-flight) and turn on the parasympathetic nervous system (rest-and-digest).

▷ Increase levels of the neurotransmitter GABA.

NOTES

1. See *Sinister Yogis* by David Gordon White for more detail on the breadth of yoga that has existed.

2. The roots of Classical Yoga go deeply into the forest and many of the practices described in the Yoga Sutra existed for centuries before the text was compiled. For more on the history of the Yoga Sutra, see Georg Feuerstein's *The Yoga Tradition*.

3. This form of disembodied liberation is known as *videha-mukti*.

4. Prakriti is everything outside of pure consciousness: everything we see, touch, feel, think, remember, or sense in any way is prakriti. From the most obvious element, earth, to the most subtle thought, emotion, sense of self (ego), or intelligence, all we can discern is prakriti.

5. We can call this a science because it meets the classic requirements of any scientific investigation; a model is posited that predicts certain testable behaviors, which can be verified by anyone who duplicates the conditions of the inquiry. The challenge is—very few people are equipped with, or can develop, the abilities to meet these conditions of inquiry.

6. *Purusha* here refers to the cosmic man or the original Self from which all comes. During the classical Yoga era, and especially in the Samkhya philosophy of that time, it came to signify our own individual consciousness, separate from all other purushas. Great debates raged over whether there were many purushas or only one great purusha, known later by various names such as brahman, Ishvara, paramatman, or one of the great gods, Vishnu or Shiva.

7. For more information on the five minor pranas, please visit www.YinYoga.com.

8. *Vayu* means "wind" or "air."

9. John Friend calls samana "muscular energy"—the drawing of the muscles to the bone—and vyana "organic energy"—the flowing of energy outward from the bones.

10. See Dr. Hiroshi Motoyama's *Theories of the Chakras*.

11. Georg Feurstein, *Shambhala Encyclopedia of Yoga*, p. 162.

12. *Vibhutis* are special powers obtained via yoga that give the yogi magic abilities.

13. The two words that make up the word "Hatha" in Hatha Yoga are *ha* and *tha*. Most teachers interpret *ha* to mean the sun and *tha* to mean the moon. However, as usual in the world of yoga, there is no unanimity. T.K.V. Desikachar in his book *The Heart of Yoga* defines *ha* to be the moon and *tha* to be the sun. But even he admits the left nostril is the lunar channel.

14. There are ways to change the flow of the breath so you won't have to tell your anxious lover to wait for a couple of hours. A sinus reflex can be stimulated, allowing the breath to switch sides within a few minutes. There are a couple of ways to tap into this reflex. One way is to lie on your side that is already open with that arm extended under your head and used as a pillow. Another approach

is to sit and shift your weight to the buttock of the open nostril. If neither intervention works, please do not blame yoga for your lover's frustration.

15. It is from this hierarchy that we derive the saying "being in seventh heaven" to signify our greatest joy.

16. Georg Feuerstein, *Tantra: The Path of Ecstasy* (Boston: Shambhala, 1998) has a good introduction to this topic. Another source that can be investigated is Joseph Campbell's *Transformation of Myth through Time* (New York: Harper Perennial, 1999).

17. See Hiroshi Motoyama, *Awakening of the Chakras and Emancipation* (Tokyo: Human Science Press, 2003). Also of interest is his book *Theory of the Chakras: Bridge to Higher Consciousness* (Wheaton, IL: Quest Books, 1988). Another good introduction to this view of energy and chakras is Paul Grilley's DVD *Chakra Theory and Meditation*.

18. In Sanskrit these blockages are known as granthis (pronounced "grunties"). You can tell from the sound of this word, you don't want grunties in your body! Granthis bad.

19. The Hatha Yoga Pradipika (2.15) warns, "Just as lions, elephants, or tigers are tamed gradually, so the life force is controlled gradually or else it will kill the practitioner himself."

20. At least initially, when immortality in this present body became rather elusive, the intention evolved into one where the practitioner sought spiritual immortality.

21. It should be noted that what we call today Traditional Chinese Medicine is not actually the original Chinese medicine! For more information on this, read Mark Seem's book *Acupuncture Imaging: Perceiving the Energy Pathways of the Body* (Rochester, VT: Healing Arts Press, 2004).

22. Our use of the term *meridian* is not a great choice. The Chinese word is *Jing-luo*, which may better be translated as a *channel*. *Jing* here means "to go through," and *luo* means "like a net," so Jing-luo is more like a network that allows Chi to flow through our body. The word *meridian* invokes a sense that the lines are imaginary, like the meridians found on our maps of the world, and don't have this sense of channeling energy.

23. A more complete introduction to Chi can be found in Ted Kaptchuk's book *The Web That Has No Weaver: Understanding Chinese Medicine* (New York: McGraw-Hill, 2000).

24. Good foods are "chi-full" foods as opposed to so much of the "chi-free" foods we consume in our typical Western diet. Fast food is chi-free. Similarly, we all know people who are chi-full and others who drain us, who are chi-free. There are chi-full and chi-free jobs, books, movies, locations, etc.

25. To be complete we would need to investigate the five subcategories of Shen: *Yi*, which means consciousness of potential; *Hun*, our non-corporeal souls; *Zhi*, our

will; *Shen* again, but this time as our spirit; and *Po*, which is our animal soul that dies when the body dies. Unfortunately, this level of investigation is beyond our scope. See Ted Kaptchuck *The Web That Has No Weaver* to learn more.

26. There used to be a belief in the West that constant worry would lead to ulcers in the stomach. Then scientists discovered the source of ulcers was a bacterium called helicobacter pylori (H. pylori). We found out that worry was not the cause of ulcers. However, in Japan, after a severe earthquake in Kobe in 1995, the incidence of ulcers skyrocketed: there was not a big increase in H. pylori in the people's stomachs, but the stress of worrying about their homes, jobs, and families made the conditions in the stomach hospitable to the bacteria, which then multiplied and caused an increase in ulcers. See the study *Peptic ulcers after the hanshin-awaji earthquake: Increased incidence of bleeding gastric ulcers* by Nobuo Aoyama et al.

27. The Chinese never developed the concept of glands but what they ascribe to weakness in the Kidneys, doctors in the West would ascribe to adrenal exhaustion.

28. Consider, as one example, alcoholics who eventually destroy their liver: many suffer from anger management problems.

29. Another name for these locations are the tan-t'iens, which we discussed in chapter 1.

30. In Thailand a similar model of energy movement evolved through a cross-fertilization of Indian and Chinese influences. The lines of energy manipulated in Thai Yoga massage are called sens. Thai massage can be considered a form of acupressure that stimulates the flow of energy along the sen lines.

31. Within these six lower-body meridians we will discover that three are more yin-like (those that run along the inner legs) and three are more yang-like: again, we see that there is yang within yin and vice versa.

32. Unfortunately, in these pictures we can't see the inside lines on Mr. Meridian Man, so it is not possible to follow these interior routes for the meridians visually.

33. See the sections on Yin Yoga for the upper body in chapter 3 and the flow for the whole body in chapter 4.

34. We discussed the practice of Nadi Shodhana in chapter 2.

35. James Oschman's book, *Energy Medicine*, has a brief but interesting review of the history of medicine and of the use of magnets and electricity by doctors in the nineteenth century.

36. The piezoelectric phenomenon has been known for over a hundred years and was given its name in 1824 by David Brewster.

37. James Oschman, *Energy Medicine in Therapeutics and Human Performance*, p. 87.

38. This is 20,000 times stronger than the cell phone.

39. If you have ever had an electrocardiogram, you may have noticed that the electrodes were placed over the heart and in more distant locations, sometimes on the ankles or wrists. These electrodes pick up the electromagnetic field of the heart as it moves out over the whole body.

40. SQUID stands for Superconducting Quantum Interference Device. Through their invention, magnetic resonance imaging (MRI) machines became possible.

41. Such as Kusaka Seto of Japan.

42. See Oschman, *Energy Medicine*, p. 78.

43. A hertz (or hz) refers to the number of times each second that the magnetic field pulsates. 30 hz means the field pulses 30 times each second. A 0.3 hz measurement means the field pulses every 3 seconds.

44. One speculation as to how these therapists could generate such large magnetic fields suggests that they were somehow tapping into the earth's own magnetic field. Interestingly, at times the therapists would lose their abilities. One possible cause for this is the ever-changing frequency of the earth's magnetic field. Normally the earth's field pulsates at something known as the Schumann's frequency, which is in the range of 7–10 Hz. However certain events like solar flares can cause the fluctuation to cease, and this may cause therapists and other Chi masters to have lesser abilities at those times.

45. See "Pulsed electromagnetic field (PEMF) treatment for fracture healing," Current Orthopaedic Practice by Boopalan, *PRJVC* et al, August 2009.

46. See Oschman's book *Energy Medicine,* chapter fourteen, for more details on this topic.

47. According to an article in *Science* (Feb 11, 2011), there are 80 billion neurons in the human brain that communicate with each other through 150 trillion synapses, which are the points of communication between cells. That's just within the brain!

48. See letters "Thumbs Up for Acupuncture" and "Thumbs Down for Acupuncture" in *Science*: November 1997 and January 1998.

49. See "Study Maps Effect of Acupuncture on the Brain" in *Science Daily*, February 2010.

50. See "Acupuncture Just as Effective Without Needle Puncture" in *Science Daily*, December 2008.

51. For a more skeptical investigation on the claims of acupuncture read The Committee for Skeptical Inquiry's report on their visit to China to investigate Traditional Chinese Medicine and acupuncture, entitled *Traditional Medicine and Pseudoscience in China* from 1996.

52. See Oschman, *Energy Medecine*, p. 77.

53. H.M. Langevin, et al., "Mechanical signaling, etc" *FASEB Journal* 15 [2001], pp. 2275-82.

54. Timothy McCall, *Yoga as Medicine: The Yogic Prescription for Health and Healing*, p. 49.

55. Ibid.

56. GABA stands for gamma aminobutyric acid.

57. C.C. Streeter, et al., "Effects of Yoga Versus Walking on Mood, Anxiety, and Brain GABA Levels: A Randomized Controlled MRS Study," *The Journal of Alternative and Complementary Medicine*, [Nov. 2010], pp. 1145-52

58. Check other issues of the *Journal of Alternative and Complementary Medicine*.

59. Heart Rate Variability (HRV) refers to the difference in heart rate that occurs as we breathe. You may think that a healthy heart keeps one beat, like a metronome, but a healthy heart speeds up as we inhale, beating faster, and slows down as we exhale. The change in rhythm is the HRV, or the RR interval as it is sometimes referred to. People with heart disease have very little HRV.

60. Our baroreflex helps to maintain our blood pressure. For example, when we suddenly stand up, the baroreflex increases our blood pressure so we don't feel faint.

61. See *British Medical Journal* [Dec. 2001] vol. 323, pp. 1446-49.

chapter eight The Heart & Mind Benefits

Remember when we talked about the three principles of the Yin Yoga practice in chapter 2? They were:

1. come into the pose to an appropriate depth

2. resolve to remain still

3. hold the pose for time

Holding the pose for time is the magic ingredient in Yin Yoga that benefits us physiologically; when we hold the stress of a pose for a long time our tissues deform, reform, and become stronger, thicker, and longer. Coming to an appropriate edge is the magic ingredient that benefits us energetically: we stimulate the acupressure points and meridian lines that send energy to our organs. Resolving to remain still is the magic ingredient that benefits us mentally and emotionally. This is our final investigation.

Look again at the yin/yang symbol here: notice once more that black, yin dot within the white, yang swirl. This is the still point. Consider a powerful, destructive hurricane: at the center is the eye—the point of absolute stillness. Think of a top spinning at high speed: at the fastest spin, the top is completely motionless. Now think of all the drama and activities happening in your life right now: where is your still point? Where do you go to find the eye of your storm?

We can practice finding the still-point at the center of our drama when we hold a Yin Yoga pose long enough that we become challenged. The urge to move is growing stronger and our mind is chattering but we continue to breathe with awareness until finally, the eye appears. The winds are still flowing furiously all around us, but we have become calm.

When we practice, finding calmness in the midst of a fierce storm during our yoga practice we learn how to find that same centered still-point at other times in our lives, when drama threatens to overwhelm us. When we are calm, our vision expands and we can decide more skillfully the course of action we wish to follow. When we are stressed, when the sympathetic nervous system is active, when our mind is frantic with thoughts, when our breath is quick, shallow, or uneven, our vision narrows: we are impelled to take the first and quickest solution in front of us. We have no ability to seek a wiser path; we simply react instead of reflect. When we practice mindfulness, at first within our yoga practice so that we learn how to also practice during the rest of our life, we learn to pause and see what is actually going on, and thus we are open to taking wiser actions.

The Benefits of Mindfulness

There have been many studies over the past few decades showing the physiological effects of mindfulness-based stress reduction (MBSR) practices.[1] Many of these we have already referred to:

 ▷ Improved blood pressure and lowered heart rate

 ▷ Reduced fight-or-flight stress response

 ▷ Activated rest-and-digest response

 ▷ Improved digestion

 ▷ Lessened inflammation

 ▷ Improved immune system

These are the physical benefits of mindfulness, and they are great! Who doesn't want a stronger immune system or better cardiovascular health? We have also seen that by paying attention to sensations and our breath we can enhance the flow of energy through our body, nourishing our organs and improving communication between cells. Mindfulness helps us physically and energetically, but we also gain from this practice emotionally.

Connecting the Dots

The heart, mind, and body are not three separate things. Scientist find it very helpful to break a system down into components in order to understand the whole; however, sometimes this classification technique requires tearing the whole apart in order to create the subsystems. The whole is always greater than the sum of the parts. To investigate the benefits of Yin Yoga emotionally and psychologically, it is useful to consider a model of the heart, mind, and body that is reconnected. Let's consider these to be three dots.

The first dot is our heart: the seat of emotions. The second is our mind: the seat of thoughts. The third dot is our body: our physical home. These three are connected: when we stimulate one of them, the others react. For example, when someone yells at us we immediately feel an emotion, perhaps of fear or maybe of anger. The emotion arises in the emotional body, which we are loosely calling our heart.[2] The emotional body quickly stimulates our physical body: we begin to secrete hormones from the adrenal glands that get us ready to fight, argue, or retreat. Our heart rate rises, we feel flushed, our pupils dilate—we are ready for some sort of action. This physical response creates certain thought patterns within our mind: we start to create thoughts about what is happening and how we are right, the other person is wrong, how unfair the situation is, etc.

Emotions stimulate the physical body, the physical body stimulates the mind, and the mind stimulates emotions. This cycle can spiral out of control in a negative feedback loop until a petty annoyance can become a towering rage. It is not possible for most of us to consciously control our adrenal glands or amygdala. It is not possible for most of us to stop strong emotions from arising. It is possible, however, for everyone to change their thoughts. We can interrupt this feedback loop by turning off the flow of negative feedback between the mind and the heart, by changing our thoughts. While this is possible, it is not easy.

Paying Attention

It is possible to change our thoughts, but to do so we first have to pay attention to them. We have to be mindful of what is actually happening right here, right now. In chapter 2 we looked at how to take an inner inventory of what we are feeling. It begins simply: pay attention to your breath that is happening right now. From here, begin to notice the sensation of breathing; notice what happens as you breathe. Next, become aware of the emotional backdrop that is present in your heart-space. Finally, become aware of your thoughts. Of course, we always have thoughts coming and going. Never are we trying to change what we were experiencing: we are simply open to whatever is arising and passing. This is the beginning of using mindfulness therapeutically, to help us in our daily life deal with the inevitable dramas that occur now and then.

There are four reactions we can have to the strong sensations that will arise in a Yin Yoga practice: two of these are yin-like and two are yang-like. Only one is really skillful; the other three occur more out of habit than by choice. The reaction we default to in our practice is most likely the reaction we also default to at other times in our lives when we face a great challenge:

1. running away from what is happening

2. trying to change what is happening

3. giving up and suffering through what is happening

4. accepting what is happening

During our Yin Yoga practice, when the drama reaches a peak, when we really want to come out, by paying attention to what is happening, we notice our cravings and our aversions. We start to notice how we want something else other than what is happening right now. Are you running away by mentally hiding in some fantasy? Are you moving to a slightly different position? Are you staying still but getting upset and thinking of how this is a stupid pose and a stupid teacher and you don't deserve to be treated like this? Or, do you accept that, at this moment in your life, this is what you are experiencing?

For some of us, our preferred response is to change the world. This is a highly valued quality in our culture. For others, our preferred response to life crises is to hide: this is the running away technique. These are both yang strategies we use to deal with challenges. The third is a yin strategy: just give up and feel sorry for ourselves: we are helpless victims.

None of these three strategies are skillful, but they are common. The final strategy is also yin-like but very skillful: paying attention and accepting what is happening. This does not mean that we continue to do nothing, if doing nothing is inappropriate. We may choose to do something, but it will be a conscious decision based upon our best judgment at that time. In a Yin Yoga pose, after five minutes, we may decide, wisely, that it is indeed time to move, but this is a conscious decision and not a default reaction to what is happening. This decision can only happen when we are mindful and paying attention to our breath, our body and our thoughts.

Dukkha

Dukkha is a Pali word that has been translated in many different ways.[3] It is used frequently in Buddhism, where it is often translated as "suffering."[4] The Buddha noted that all life contains three characteristics—*dukkha, anicca,* and *anatta*: suffering, impermanence, and no independent arising or self. Dukkha is part of life: if you are alive you will experience it.

A better translation of the word could be *unsatisfactoriness* or *unreliableness.* Life is not always sorrowful or filled with suffering, but there are times when pain will arise, when things will happen that we wish were not happening. That is dukkha. How we react is what creates our suffering and sorrow. Pain is just pain: when we make a drama around it, we turn the pain into suffering.

The difference between pain and suffering is nicely illustrated through a parable that the Buddha once related. One day the Buddha was sitting in front of a group of monks and he asked them, "Imagine there was a man, and imagine that this man had just been shot in the thigh with an arrow: how would the man feel?" The monks replied, "Hurt! In pain!" "Right," said the Buddha, "Now, imagine that this man got hit by a second arrow, right in the same spot! Now how would he feel?" "Worse! Agony!" responded the monks. "Exactly," said the Buddha, "And the name of that second arrow is suffering ... and it is optional!"

The first of the Buddha's two arrows is dukkha: there will be times in life when pain arises. The second arrow, which he called suffering, is caused by what we do about the first arrow, and that is why it is optional. We could choose to just be with the pain that has arisen in our life, but we don't: we add to it. We love to create drama. A comedian once said that Christmas is a time when dysfunctional families get back together and retraumatize the hell out of each other. This is optional!

The Buddha is famous for being the first, but not the last, to point out that we are what we think. If we allow our thoughts to linger negatively on what is happening, or worse, if we allow our thoughts to remain negatively on what might happen or what has happened, we are striking ourselves with that second arrow. If you want to be unhappy, think about unhappy things. If you want to be content, think of all the things you already have.[5] This may seem, on the surface, to be a variation of the first strategy described earlier, of running away or ignoring what is happening, but it's really the last strategy: we pay attention to what is actually happening, notice what our reaction is, evaluate whether this reaction is a wise one or not, and if not, change it by changing our thoughts.

What does this have to do with our Yin Yoga practice? It is during Yin Yoga that we get to practice this advanced level of paying attention to our life. When we are at our edge and feeling the juiciness of the pose, we are simulating a challenging time. Now we get to notice our habitual pattern of reaction, and if it is not skillful, work to change that reaction, to create a new pattern.

Pathing

Pop quiz: what is the difference between being stuck in a rut and being in the groove? People hate being stuck in a rut, doing the same old same old everyday. But, being in the groove means you're on a roll. Athletes call it being in the zone: they practice the same motions over and over again until they become automatic. Dancers and musicians similarly want to find that place where they can just flow. The only difference between a rut and a groove is our attitude toward what we are doing: if we don't like what we are doing, it's a rut but if we love what we are doing, we're in the groove.

Our habitual patterns are paths: we can call them grooves or ruts depending upon whether they serve us well or not. There is an ancient concept called karma that embodies this: our current actions are the results of our past actions. This is exactly how a path is created. To illustrate, think of a beautiful forest: imagine that you want to get from one side to the other, and you are the first person or animal to have ever traversed these woods. It is not easy to walk through virgin forests: you have to blaze a trail. The first time you walk the trail it is hard work. You may have to carve out your path. The second time you do it, it is a bit easier. After walking this path 100 times, it is really easy to follow the trail and difficult to leave the path to go in another direction. To go somewhere else requires blazing a new path, with all that effort being redone.

It is no wonder that people stick to their ruts in life: it is hard to create a new path. Athletes and musicians have to work very hard to blaze the new paths in their neural networks so that their performance is easy. But, if the path you are following is no longer serving you, get off that path and blaze a new one! Our thoughts create paths in our brains, as well. It is not easy to stop thinking in the same old ways we have always thought. If your standard strategy for dealing with challenges in life is number one, two, or three above, you have created a path that will be difficult to change—but far from impossible!

Yin Yoga is the chance to practice changing our chosen paths: we get to blaze new trails, more skillful grooves to follow. Again, the process is quite simple: notice what is going on, choose not to default to your habitual response, consider what is the most skillful thing to do right now, and then do it.

Watering Flowers

Watering is an excellent metaphor to illustrate how we default to following a path in our mind that does not serve us well. As we become more practiced at noticing our thoughts and emotional states, we will discover that we spend a lot of time watering weeds. Now, if you are a gardener you'd think this was a very silly thing to do. Don't water weeds: water the flowers! But the path to the weed patch is well worn from years of walking there. It is easy to get to the weed patch, so we allow our thinking to just go to these weeds.

What are the weeds in your mind's garden? Whenever you allow thoughts of regret, fear, anxiety, anger, frustration, envy, jealousy, sadness, or guilt to linger you are watering weeds. Whenever you allow your thoughts to remain on things long past that you wished had turned out differently, or fantasize about a future that you know cannot be, you are watering weeds. And, of course, the more you water these weeds, the taller and pricklier they become. The more you walk the path to the weed patch, the easier it is to continue to go there. Yin Yoga gives you the chance to stop watering your weeds and start watering your flowers!

Remember: it is not easy to get out of a rut, but it is possible. When you notice that your mind is thinking about weeds, take your watering can and go over to your flower garden: start watering your flowers. It takes a while to build a new habit and stop an old one. It requires intention and attention: remember why you are doing this! Use the power of your intention to give you the strength to get out of that old mental rut and blaze a new path to your garden.

When you have left the weed patch, you can direct your mind to linger on thoughts of joy, compassion, kindness, equanimity, and love. Everyone has flowers to water: if you have difficulty with this practice, start with the beautiful flower of gratitude. Bring to your mind all the things in your life that you are so grateful for. Once you start thinking about gratitude, you will discover so many flowers all around you: think of your parents, your children, your friends, your health.[6] You can meditate on how grateful you are for your job, your home, your city or country, for the hobbies in your life that give you so much pleasure, your books and music, for sports and for the great outdoors, to be able to learn new things, and of course, you can think about how grateful you are for your yoga practice.

If you cannot think of any flower to water right now, a flower that is always with you is your breath: be grateful for this breath that you are breathing right now. Enjoy your breath. Watch your breath. Simply by returning to the flower of this breath, you stop watering weeds. When we stop watering our weeds, they dry up and wither. When you stop visiting the weed patch, the path eventually becomes overgrown and hard to follow, while the path to your flower garden becomes easier and easier to follow. Eventually, we no longer go to the weed patch: it is so much easier and more enjoyable to go water our lovely flowers.

Mindfulness

Mindfulness simply means to pay attention: this is the practice of presence. During our yoga practice, we build the habit of mindfulness so that we can call upon this skill at any time that we need presence. Thich Nhat Hanh, a world-renowned teacher of engaged Buddhism and mindfulness, explains it this way:

> Mindfulness is the energy of being aware and awake to the present moment. It is the continuous practice of touching life deeply in every moment. To be mindful is to be truly alive and at one with those around us. Practicing mindfulness does not require that we go anywhere different.
>
> We can practice mindfulness in our room and on our way from one place to another. We can do very much the same things we always do— walking, sitting, working, eating, talking—except we learn to do them with an awareness of what we are doing.[7]

This is the goal when we hold yin poses in stillness: we awaken to the present moment. We touch what is happening in our body, and in our heart and mind. We don't have to go anywhere: right here, right now—this is life.

Summary of Heart and Mind Benefits

The act of practicing presence, of being mindful of what is happening right now, can help us physiologically, energetically, and mentally/emotionally. Our stress begins to evaporate as soon as we pay attention to our breath and allow it to slow down. When our stress level declines we reap many health benefits: our blood pressure drops, heart rate slows, immune system reactivates, digestion improves, and inflammation decreases. By paying attention to the sensations within, we can stimulate and enhance energy movement. And, by being present, we can choose to change our brain.

We all have habitual reactions to life that we no longer think about. These are unconscious reactions that may have served us well at one time, but are no longer the best choices we could make today. Since we are not conscious of these reactions, we don't stop to think about how we could do better: we simply live life the way we always have. But, if we are finding that life is not as satisfying as it could be or once was, perhaps it is time to take a deeper look at how we are responding to life. Instead of life being something that is just happening, we can discover that we are free to build new, skillful habits that will enhance our enjoyment of life. We do this through mindfulness, which we develop through the stillness of our yoga practice.

In Yin Yoga we come to an edge in a pose and become still. While we hold the pose, we go within. We start to notice what is going on in life, right here, right now—without adding any drama, without taking anything away from the experience. With clarity we see what is really needed, beyond the cravings and aversions that normally move us. We are now free to create a new response, and over time build new paths to follow.

The real benefits of yoga are physical, emotional, and mental health and well-being. We build habits that last a lifetime. We become present and enjoy this moment, the moment that is happening right now. We become grateful for this wonderful gift—and perhaps we resolve to share what we have discovered with others, so that they, too, can live life well.

NOTES

1. For a complete investigation into MBSR benefits, check out the work of John Kabat-Zinn.

2. In this map, we are not dividing the home of our emotions into all the major organs as the Daoist maps do. Nor are we looking at the centers in the brain, such as the amygdala, which scientists know starts the chain of reactions when we are frightened. We are proposing a much simpler model here, in which we see all emotions arising in the heart.

3. In Sanskrit it is written *duhkha*. Since the original Buddhist texts were written in Pali, we are using the Pali spelling.

4. The original use of the word referred to the center of a wheel, such as a potter's wheel or a chariot wheel. If the center was not quite centered, the wheel did not spin well: that was dukkha. If the center was right in the middle of the wheel, the wheel spun nicely: this is called *sukha*, which is often translated as *happiness*.

5. Rabbi Schwartz once said, "True happiness is wanting what you already have." That's a quick way to contentment.

6. Even if your health is relatively poor right now, it could still be far worse! Be grateful for what you do have.

7. From *Happiness: Essential Mindfulness Practices* by Thich Nhat Hanh.

BIBLIOGRAPHY

Alter, Michael. *The Science of Flexibility* (Champaign, IL: Human Kinetics, 2004).

Becker, Robert O. and Marino, Andrew A. *Electromagnetism and Life* (StonyBrook, NY: SUNY Press, 1982).

Campbell, Joseph. *Transformation of Myth Through Time* (New York: Harper Perennial, 1999).

Desikachar, T. K. V. *Health, Healing and Beyond* (New York: North Point Press, 1998).

Doniger, Wendy. trans., *Rig Veda* (New York: Penguin, 1981).

Feuerstein, Georg. *Tantra: The Path of Ecstasy* (Boston: Shambhala, 1998).

———. *The Yoga Sutra* (Rochester, VT: Inner Traditions, 1989).

———. *The Yoga Tradition: Its History, Literature, Philosophy and Practice* (Prescott, AZ: Hohm Press, 2001).

———. *The Shambhala Encyclopedia of Yoga* (Boston: Shambhala, 2000).

Freeman, Richard. *The Yoga Matrix Audio CD* (Boulder, CO: Sounds True, 2003).

Grilley, Paul. *Anatomy of Yoga DVD* (San Francisco: Pranamaya, 2008).

———. *Yin Yoga: Outline of a Quiet Practice* (Ashland, OR: White Cloud Press, 2002).

Hedley, Gil. *The Integral Anatomy Series*, vols. 1-4 (Beverly Hills, FL: Integral Anatomy Productions, 2005-2009.

Holt, L., Pelham, T., and Holt, J. *Flexibility: A Concise Guide* (Humana Press, 2008).

Iyengar, B. K. S. *Light on Yoga: Yoga Dipika* (New York: Schocken Books, 1979).

Johnson, Robert. *Owning Your Own Shadow: Understanding the Dark Side of the Psyche* (New York: HarperCollins, 1993).

Jois, Sri K. Pattabhi. *Yoga Mala: The Original Teachings of Ashtanga Yoga Master Sri K. Pattabhi Jois* (New York: North Point Press, 2000).

Kaptchuk, Ted. *The Web That Has No Weaver: Understanding Chinese Medicine* (New York: McGraw-Hill, 2000).

Lindsay, Mark. *Fascia: Clinical Applications for Health and Human Performance* (Clifton Park, NY: Delmar Cengage Learning, 2008).

Mallinson, James. *The Gheranda Samhita* (Woodstock, NY: YogaVidya.com, 2004).

———. trans., *Shiva Samhita* (Woodstock, NY: YogaVidya.com, 2007).

McCall, Timothy. *Yoga as Medicine: The Yogic Prescription for Health and Healing* (New York: Bantam Books, 2007).

McGill, Stuart. *Low Back Disorders* (Champaign, IL: Human Kinetics, 2002).

Mohan, A. G. *Krishnamacharya: His Life and Teachings* (Boston: Shambhala, 2010).

Motoyama, Hiroshi. *Awakening of the Chakras and Emancipation* (Tokyo: Human Science Press, 2003).

———. *Measurements of Ki Energy, Diagnosis, and Treatments* (Encinitas, CA: California Institute for Human Science, 1997).

———. *Theory of the Chakras: Bridge to Higher Consciousness* (Wheaton, IL: Quest Books, 1988).

Oschman, James. *Energy Medicine: the Scientific Basis* (Philadelphia: Churchill Livingston, 2000).

———. *Energy Medicine in Therapeutics and Human Performance* (Waltham, MA: Butterworth-Heinemann, 2003).

Powers, Sarah, *Insight Yoga* (Boston: Shambhala, 2008).

———. *Insight Yoga DVD* (San Francisco: Pranamaya, 2005).

Seem, Mark. *Acupuncture Imaging: Perceiving the Energy Pathways of the Body* (Rochester, VT: Healing Arts Press, 2004).

Strom, Max. *A Life Worth Breathing: A Yoga Master's Handbook of Strength, Grace, and Healing* (New York: Skyhorse Publishing, 2010).

Swatmarama, Swami. *Hatha Yoga Pradīpika* (Seattle, WA: Pacific Publishing Studio, 2011).

Thich Nhat Hanh. *Happiness: Essential Mindfulness Practices* (Berkeley: Parallax Press, 2009).

White, David Gordon. *Sinister Yogis* (Chicago: University of Chicago Press, 2009).

Wilhelm, Richard. *Tao Te Ching* (New York: Prentice Hall, 2002).

———. *The Secret of the Golden Flower* (New York: Harcourt & Brace, 1962).

Wong, Eva. *The Shambhala Guide to Taoism Yoga* (Boston: Shambhala, 1996).

———. *Taoism: An Essential Guide* (Boston: Shambhala, 2011).

INDEX

About the Author

Bernie has been teaching yoga and meditation since 1998. He has a bachelors degree in Science from the University of Waterloo and combines his intense interest in yoga with an understanding of the scientific approach to investigating the nature of things. His ongoing studies have taken him deeply inside mythology, comparative religions, and psychology. All of these avenues of exploration have clarified his understanding of the ancient Eastern practices of yoga and meditation. His teaching, workshops and books have helped many students broaden their own understanding of health, life and the source of true joy.

Bernie's yoga practice encompasses the hard, yang-styles, such as Ashtanga and Power Yoga, as well as the softer, yin-styles, as exemplified in Yin Yoga. His meditation experience goes back to the early 80's when he first began to explore the practice of Zen meditation. During those days, while he struggled with the conflict between practice and theory, Bernie also worked as a member of the executive team of one of Canada's oldest and largest high technology companies. He lives in Vancouver, British Columbia.

For more information on Bernie, visit www.yinyoga.com

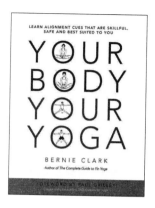

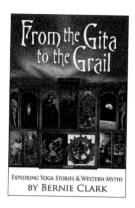

Your Body, Your Yoga

Learn Alignment Cues That Are Skillful, Safe, and Best Suited To You

Your Body, Your Yoga goes beyond any prior yoga anatomy book available. It looks not only at the body's unique anatomical structures and what this means to everyone's individual range of motion, but also examines the physiological sources of restrictions to movement.

"*Your Body, Your Yoga* is a fascinating, provocative, and scientifically-informed look at the inner workings of the body as it affects the practice of asana. Bernie Clark challenges much dogma in the modern postural yoga world, including a few heretofore sacrosanct principles of alignment, to demonstrate that a healthy and effective yoga practice should be adapted to each individual's unique needs, abilities and anatomy. Required reading for yoga teachers and yoga therapists, and highly recommended for avid practitioners."
—*Timothy McCall, MD, author of Yoga As Medicine; U.S.A.*

From The Gita to The Grail

Exploring Yoga Stories & Western Myths

Learn what the myths of yoga mean to those of us who grew up in Western culture and with Western stories.

"In this insightful book, Bernie reminds us that we have a choice in how we live our lives; we can hold tight to our beliefs, allowing them to dictate our reality, or we can invite every story (or even encounter) to be a gateway into the poetic, multifaceted dimensions of truth, and the fluid nature of reality."
—*Sarah Powers, author of Insight Yoga and founder of the Insight Yoga Institute*

"Bernie's book covers mythical territory any student of yoga should be aware of. Diving into both unfamiliar and familiar stories of creation and the path of the hero, Bernie's readable style is like the voice of an Elder. If you could record Joseph Campbell and Carl Jung's conversation over a game of chess, it might sound something like this."
—*Daniel Clement, founder of Open Source Yoga*